The
Nautilus
Book

The Nautilus Book

An Illustrated Guide to Physical Fitness the Nautilus Way

Ellington Darden, Ph.D.

Contemporary Books, Inc.
Chicago

Library of Congress Cataloging in Publication Data

Darden, Ellington, 1943–
  The Nautilus book.

  Includes index.
  1. Weight lifting.   2. Weight lifting—Equipment
and supplies.   3. Physical fitness.   I. Title.
GV546.D28   1980   796.4′1′028   80-10471
ISBN 0-8092-7100-1
ISBN 0-8092-7099-4 pbk.

Copyright © 1980 by Ellington Darden
All rights reserved
Published by Contemporary Books, Inc.
180 North Michigan Avenue, Chicago, Illinois 60601
Manufactured in the United States of America
Library of Congress Catalog Card Number: 80-10471
International Standard Book Number: 0-8092-7100-1 (cloth)
                                    0-8092-7099-4 (paper)

Published simultaneously in Canada by
Beaverbooks
953 Dillingham Road
Pickering, Ontario L1W 1Z7
Canada

contents

acknowledgments

The author would like to thank Lona Dion, Casey Viator, Scott LeGear, and Don Litwin for their part in this book. Lona and Casey demonstrated the Nautilus exercises for the able camera of Scott LeGear. Scott's artistic photographs not only enhance the book, but also serve as an excellent means of instructing people in the proper use of each Nautilus machine. Don Litwin read the manuscript and made valuable contributions.

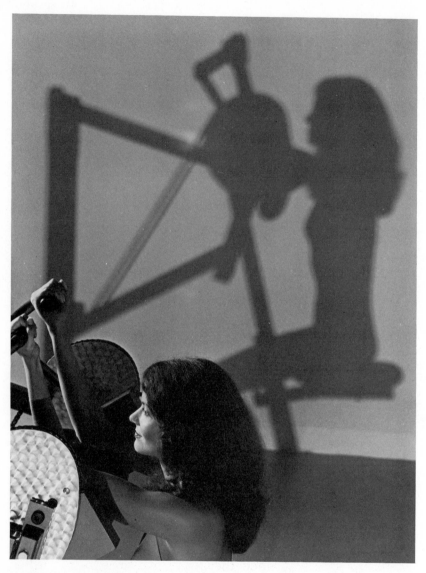

Multi-biceps machine

introduction

In 1970, after 20 years of experimentation, Arthur Jones built and sold an exercise machine. It was a pullover machine for the torso muscles. This was the first tool on the market to provide variable resistance. The resistance was varied by the use of carefully designed eccentric cams, or spiral pulleys.

As Jones was studying the spiral pulleys, it occurred to him that they resembled a cross section of the chambered nautilus shell. The chambered nautilus is a mollusk which, because of its geometric perfection, has survived at the bottom of the Pacific Ocean for millions of years. It was an ideal symbol for the new machines. A year later, the new company in Lake Helen, Florida, became Nautilus Sports/Medical Industries. Since then, Nautilus exercise machines have revolutionized the concept of training and conditioning the human body.

The reason Nautilus revolutionized physical conditioning was, in one word, efficiency. Nautilus training was much

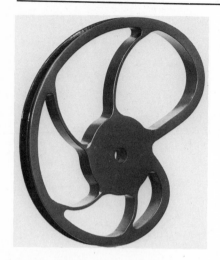 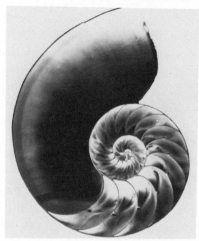

Arthur Jones's original spiral pulleys reminded him of a cross section of the chambered nautilus shell; so he named his new exercise machines Nautilus.

more efficient than traditional methods of exercise. Earlier methods of conditioning had centered around long programs of exercise. To obtain a high level of fitness, an individual had to spend a minimum of 90 minutes a day on stretching for flexibility, jogging for heart-lung endurance, and lifting barbells for strength. The average fitness enthusiast might spend from 5 to 10 hours a week on such exercise programs.

If Nautilus machines required the same amount of time as traditional methods and produced slightly better results, that would still be a worthwhile contribution. But if Nautilus machines produced three times the results in *one-tenth* of the time, that could only be described as revolutionary. And that is exactly what Nautilus produced: three times the results in one-tenth of the time!

Nautilus machines first gained publicity in the bodybuilding field. After being trained by Arthur Jones and his machines for six months, 19-year-old Casey Viator, who demonstrated some of the exercises in this book, won the 1971 Mr. America contest with obvious ease. Not only did he win the main title, but he took all the awards for body parts with the exception of best abdominals. He remains the youngest man ever to win the title. His victory in the Mr. America contest attracted the attention of football coaches to Nautilus strength-building machines. Soon, Nautilus was being used for football conditioning. In 1972, the Miami Dolphins were the first National Football League team to incorporate Nautilus into their conditioning program. The Cincinnati Bengals followed suit, as did the Houston Oilers and the Buffalo Bills. Now 27 of the 28 teams have the equipment.

The National Football League's use of Nautilus machines gave considerable credibility to their effectiveness. Now other sports teams such as basketball, hockey, baseball, wrestling, and swimming employ Nautilus in their training programs.

This interest naturally aroused the attention of the fitness and health centers that catered to millions of non-athletes across the nation. As Nautilus effectiveness was demonstrated, more and more fitness centers began ordering full sets of Nautilus. Nautilus fitness centers began to spring up in all major cities. By the end of 1979, there were over 1,300 fitness centers using Nautilus equipment.

Today, the sale of Nautilus equipment to fitness centers represents only about a third of the machines sold. Nautilus machines are used by sports medicine clinics, hospitals, rehabilitation centers, law enforcement agencies, the armed forces, professional sports teams, colleges, high schools, corporate recreation centers, exercise physiology laboratories, racquetball and tennis clubs, and private individuals. Such sales are not only national, but international.

Having access to Nautilus machines is merely the initial step in obtaining superior results from exercise. Using Nautilus equipment correctly is of equal importance. Function dictates design, and each Nautilus machine was designed according to the physiological functions of the human body. An understanding and application of the guidelines presented in this book will allow you to obtain the best possible results from Nautilus training.

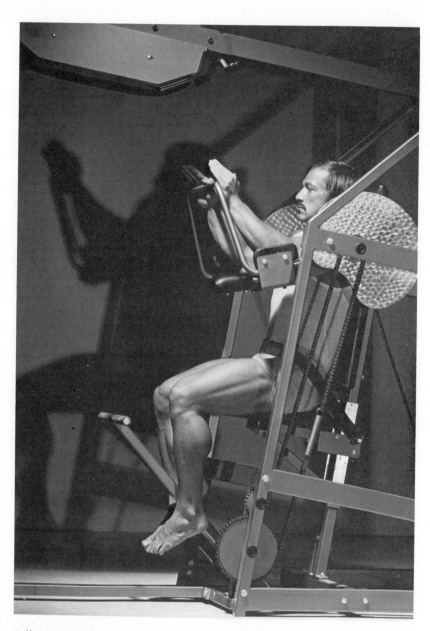

Pullover/torso arm machine

CHAPTER ONE

the requirements of full-range exercise

Most exercise books urge you to practice full-range movements. Such advice is largely wasted, because full-range movement against resistance is impossible in most conventional exercises.

A barbell curl is not a full-range exercise. There is no resistance during the last part of the movement, no stretching is provided at the start of the movement, and there is no resistance in the finishing position.

Neither is a barbell bench press a full-range exercise, and for many of the same reasons. There is little stretching in the bottom position. The arms lock out under the weight in the top position, causing the resistance to be supported by the bones and ensuring that no work for the muscles occurs at that point.

Almost all conventional exercises suffer from similar limitations. You're trying the impossible when you attempt to provide your muscles with full-range exercise while exposing them to a straight line of resistance.

1

Muscular contraction produces a rotary movement of the related body part. The muscle contracts in an approximately straight line and produces straight-line force as a source of power. But this straight-line force is converted to a rotary form of movement by the articulation of the joint. Muscles move in straight lines, but the movement of body parts is rotary.

For most of the last 80 years, people have been trying to force their muscles to work within a framework of limitations imposed by an imperfect tool, the barbell; or by exercise machines designed to duplicate the functions of a barbell. You certainly can exercise with a barbell, but you just as certainly cannot achieve *full-range* exercise with it.

What is the importance of full-range exercise? Simply that without it, you can work no more than part of a muscle. And you cannot build a maximum level of strength and fitness exercising part of a muscle while utterly ignoring other portions of the same muscle.

Full-range exercise has 10 basic requirements. All 10 of the requirements are equally important. If any one is missing, full-range movement is impossible.

The requirements for full-range exercise are as follows:

 1. Positive Work
 2. Negative Work
 3. Rotary-Form Movement
 4. Stretching
 5. Pre-Stretching
 6. Automatically Variable Resistance
 7. Balanced Resistance
 8. Direct Resistance
 9. Resistance in the Position of Full-Muscular Contraction
10. Unrestricted Speed of Movement

Years ago, Arthur Jones set out to design and build a truly full-range exercise machine. But until he could identify the

10 basic requirements, he could not design the desired tool.

After finally determining the actual requirements for full-range exercise, Jones incorporated all of them into his Nautilus machines. Once you understand each of the requirements, you'll clearly see why exercise performed on Nautilus machines is superior to other forms of movement.

POSITIVE WORK

When you lift a weight, you're performing positive work. Your muscles are producing movement by concentric contraction, reducing their length.

Almost all forms of exercise involve positive work, even if movement of the resistance is not produced. But some forms of exercise have only positive work.

Within the last several years, much has been claimed for a form of exercise called isokinetics. But this form is limited to positive work, and all such exercises are based on friction of one kind or another.

A positive-only style of training could be produced with a barbell in either one of two ways: (1) If you lifted a barbell, immediately dropped it upon reaching the top position of movement, then lifted it again, then dropped it again, you would be exercising in a positive-only fashion. (2) If, with the help of assistants, you lifted the barbell, and if they took it from you as soon as it reached the top position and lowered it back down for you, you would be performing only the positive part of the work while the assistants performed the negative part of the work.

Such a style of training with a barbell would be very dangerous in the first instance, and impractical in the second. It would be only slightly effective in either case because a positive-only form of exercise is lacking several of the requirements for productive exercise. Positive work is certainly of value in exercise, but positive-only exercise suffers from numerous limitations.

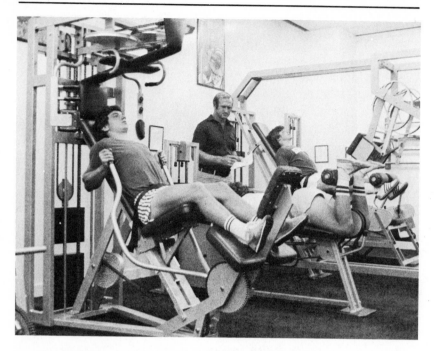

Nautilus machines provide both positive and negative work potential on each repetition.

NEGATIVE WORK

When you lower a weight, you're performing negative work. Your muscles are limiting movement by eccentric contraction, while increasing their length.

If a barbell is dropped from the top position, then negative work is not performed. Instead, the normal downward movement of the resistance that is produced by gravity must be limited. Normal acceleration must be prevented; movement must be slowed and controlled.

A negative-only style of training can be provided in several ways: (1) by assistants who lift the weight for you, so that you can limit your efforts to slowly lowering the weight, (2) by climbing on a chair into the top position of a chinning exercise, you can limit the exercise to a negative-only style by lowering yourself from the top position, or (3) by using a mechanical arrangement that lifts the weight so that you can lower it. The first style is impractical, because of the need for helpers. The second is limited to certain exercises: chinning, dipping, and a few others. The third style requires special equipment.

But do note that the negative part of movement is one of the most important parts of exercise. In fact, it is probably the most important part performed for the purpose of increasing strength. To the degree that it is possible under the prevailing circumstances, the negative part of exercise should be given as much emphasis as possible.

Many people make the mistake of paying close attention to the positive part of their exercises, but ignore the negative part. They lift the weight smoothly and in good form, then lower it in a haphazard manner. Thus, they deny themselves a large part of the potential benefits of their exercises. What you should do instead is lift the weight in a smooth steady motion, without pause and without jerking or sudden movement. Then, lower the weight in the same fashion, smoothly, steadily, and even more slowly.

Negative work is only possible when there is a source of back pressure, a force pulling in a direction opposite to the direction of movement produced by muscular contraction. During barbell exercises the muscles are pulling up and the force of gravity is pulling down. So a barbell can provide both positive and negative work.

But the friction-based type of exercise, isokinetics, does not provide negative work. There is no back pressure of force pulling the muscles back toward the starting position. In such exercises resistance is provided only while you're moving in a positive direction. If movement stops, the resistance stops.

Lacking back pressure for negative work, such exercises consequently also fail to fill several other requirements for productive exercises. Prior to the start of movement, there is no back presssure or force to pull the joints into a stretched position, and no force to pre-stretch the muscles before the start of contraction. Thus isokinetic exercise does nothing for flexibility. Flexibility requires stretching. Neither does isokinetic exercise provide a high intensity of muscular contraction, which also requires pre-stretching.

ROTARY-FORM MOVEMENT

Muscular contraction occurs in an approximately straight line, and straight-line force is produced. But the body part that is moved by muscular contraction does not move in a straight line. Instead, the body part rotates, as it must, since it is working around the axis of a joint.

The articulation of the joints converts the straight-line force of muscular contraction into the rotary-form force required for movement. Much the same thing occurs in an engine when the crankshaft converts the straight-line power produced by the cylinders into the rotary-form power required by the wheels.

When the hamstring muscles contract, the lower legs move in a rotary fashion around the knee joints. For full-range exercise of the hamstrings, the knee joints must be on a common axis with the source of resistance.

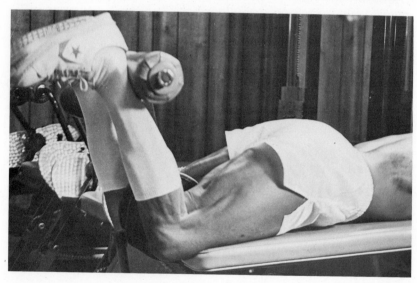

Most forms of exercise provide resistance in only one direction. This direction may be down as a result of the force of gravity during barbell exercises. It may be up (or across) during Universal machine exercises, where the resistance is redirected by the use of pulleys or levers. Or, it may be in any possible direction during isokinetic-type exercises. But in all three cases, one factor remains constant: resistance is provided in only one direction, straight-line direction.

Obviously, full-range exercise cannot co-exist with straight-line resistance, since the body part involved is constantly changing its direction of movement by rotation. Resistance, therefore, is only provided at the start of an exercise movement, during the mid-range of movement, or at the end. It is not present throughout a movement.

Resistance is provided only when the direction of movement is opposed to the direction of the pull of the resistance. That is impossible when a person is trying to apply a straight-line source of resistance against a rotary-form movement. During a barbell curl, for instance, there is no resistance at all at the start of the movement. The resistance is pulling down while the movement is forward. Thus the resistance is 90 degrees out of phase with the direction of movement.

Shortly after the curling movement is started, the direction of movement changes to the point that the resistance is almost 90 degrees out of phase with the direction of movement. At this point, some resistance is provided, but not much. That's because you're still pushing the weight more than you're lifting it.

Actually, you're lifting the weight only in one small area of movement, at the point where your hands are going straight up, while the resistance is pulling straight down. This is the so-called sticking point of the curl, where the weight feels far heavier than it does during any other part of a curl. Of course, the barbell is no heavier at that point than it is at any other point throughout the movement. But its direction of pull is exactly 180 degrees out-of-phase with the direction of movement, so it feels heavier. Once past that point, the pull of resistance rapidly drops off, and near the end of the movement, it becomes nearly zero.

The weight seems to change during a curl. This apparent change is a result of challenging a rotary movement with a straight-line source of resistance. The biceps muscles, the muscles worked during a curl, receive heavy resistance only during a very limited part of the movement. But during the rest of the movement, the resistance is far too light.

For full-range exercise, the body part that is being moved by muscular contraction must be rotating on a common axis with the source of resistance. In effect, the joint, the elbow joint in the case of a curl, must be in line with the axis of a rotary form of resistance. When this arrangement of axis points is correct, the resistance is always exactly 180 degrees out-of-phase with the momentary direction of movement. You are always *lifting* the weight, regardless of your actual direction of movement.

Without such rotary-form resistance, full-range exercise is not possible. And Nautilus training provides that resistance.

STRETCHING

A relaxed arm does not hang in a fully straightened position. It tends to remain slightly bent. The biceps that bend the arm and the triceps that straighten the arm are always pulling slightly in opposite directions.

You can straighten your arm by contracting the triceps while attempting to relax the biceps as much as possible. But you cannot stretch the biceps without an external source of force, force external to the arm itself.

If such stretching is not a regular part of your exercises, you'll gradually reduce your degree of flexibility. At the same time, you'll lose the ability to move into positions that were previously possible.

Young children are normally very flexible, but as they grow older they lose much of that flexibility. This is partially

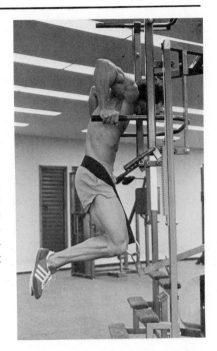

One of the best exercises for stretching and strengthening the pectoralis major muscles of the chest is the dip performed on the Nautilus multi-exercise machine. Additional resistance can be attached to the belt around the trainee's waist.

unavoidable, since some of a child's flexibility results from the fact that his bones are soft and his limbs are fairly thin. Both are factors which change with age. But a certain part of the flexibility loss that occurs between childhood and maturity is the direct result of a lack of stretching. Some of the thousands of athletic injuries that happen every year are caused by the unnatural loss of normal flexibility.

A low level of strength can be maintained with no systematic exercise. An apparently normal range of movement can also be maintained without exercise. But losses in both strength and flexibility will steadily progress without exercise, until suddenly that person finds himself to be far weaker and much less flexible than he had ever suspected.

Some barbell exercises improve flexibility, and some do not, depending on the degree of stretching involved. Exercises performed on a Universal machine generally provide less stretching than similar barbell exercises, primarily because the resistance is supported in the starting position. And isokinetic exercises do absolutely nothing for flexibility, because there is no stretching.

PRE-STRETCHING

Stretching is primarily related to the joints, muscles, and the connective tissue, but pre-stretching is related to the muscle itself. Pre-stretching is commonly known as reflex action.

When a muscle is contracted from a relaxed starting position, the resulting contraction is not as strong as it could be. That is because all of the fibers in a muscle do not contract at the same time, regardless of the amount of resistance. A muscle will fail under a load that it could move if all of the fibers were involved at the same time, and it will fail with most of the fibers still relaxed.

Pre-stretching is required for the high intensity of muscular contraction you need. If your muscle is pre-stretched prior to contraction, then it will involve a higher percentage of its fibers in the following contraction. The act of pre-stretching a muscle sends a signal to your brain that results in a higher-than-normal intensity of contraction. A center in your brain is warned in advance that the load is heavy and that as many as possible of the available fibers will be needed.

Barbell and Universal machine exercises provide this essential pre-stretching in proportion to the amount of stretching involved. So some barbell and some Universal exercises provide pre-stretching, and some do not. Isokinetic exercises do not provide pre-stretching, since they offer no negative work.

AUTOMATICALLY VARIABLE RESISTANCE

Muscles are not equally strong in all positions, and movement produces changes in the mechanical efficiency of the involved joints. As a result of these two factors, you're much stronger in some positions than you are in others. If the resistance remains constant in all positions, it will be correct in only one position and too light in all other positions throughout a full range of possible movement.

You're actually limited to the amount of resistance that you can handle in your weakest position. If you try to use more resistance, you'll find it impossible to move it through the weakest area of movement.

In practice, some variation in available resistance occurs in almost all exercises, even though the actual weight of the resistance remains constant. In that barbell curl we discussed earlier, there is no available resistance in either the starting or finishing position of the exercise. There is also a constant change in resistance as the movement occurs, since the arms moving the resistance change in relation to gravity. But such variations in resistance are random in nature, and have no relationship to the ability of the muscles to handle resistance in a particular position.

If a rotary-form curling machine is built with a round pulley directly in line with the elbow joints, the resistance will remain exactly the same throughout the full range of possible movement. It will not feel the same, however. Instead, we noted, it will feel very heavy at the start of the movement. Once moving, the weight seems to become lighter. Later in the movement, it will seem ridiculously light. Finally, at the end of the movement, the weight will begin to feel heavier again. All this is illusory, and not based on the simple facts of muscle physiology.

The resistance in a barbell curl starts at zero, then increases rapidly to peak resistance after 90 degrees of movement. It then plummets back to zero near the end of the curl. The resistance in a barbell curl, then, starts off too low, increases too rapidly, then ceases too soon.

Changing from a barbell curl to a rotary-form curling machine does not solve the problem. The level of resistance in the various positions throughout the movement is still not in accord with the available strength in the same positions. In a barbell curl, the available resistance changes, but it changes too fast, and too much. In a rotary-form curling machine, the resistance does not change at all, and it should.

The problem of these extremes is solved by the Nautilus cam. Instead of a round pulley, Nautilus machines use a spiral pulley, so that the resistance changes instantly and automatically as a movement occurs and available strength changes. Physics and muscle physiology, therefore, dictated the design of the Nautilus cams.

At the start of a curl in a Nautilus biceps curling machine, the radius of the pulley is fairly small. In that position, you're not as strong as you will be later in the movement. The machine gives you a mechanical advantage in that position. As you move into a stronger position, the radius of the pulley changes, becoming larger or smaller as it must to accommodate the level of strength available in every position.

BALANCED RESISTANCE

Having automatically variable resistance is not enough. The resistance must be varied and, in effect, balanced in accordance with your available strength in all positions.

The exact size and shape of the cam is crucially important. It must provide as much resistance in every position as you can handle in that position, but no more. While several small companies are now illegally trying to copy the Nautilus cams, so far they do not have even an elementary understanding of the cam's required shape. Having a cam is not enough. It must be the right cam for the particular application. Fords and Chevrolets both have cams. But a Chevrolet cam will not survive in a Ford, or vice versa.

So cams, correctly designed for each large muscle group, are required to balance the resistance in relation to any particular person's available strength.

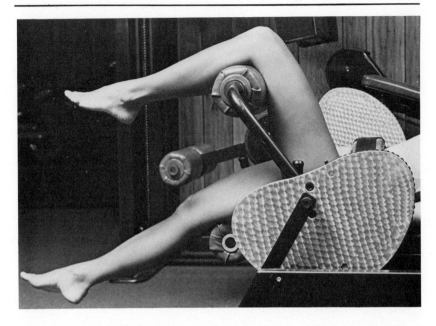

The patented Nautilus cam provides automatically variable and balanced resistance for each machine. As the radius of the cam varies, the effective resistance changes to accommodate the trainee's potential strength in all positions.

DIRECT RESISTANCE

Muscular contraction produces direct movement of the body part to which the muscle is attached. During a curl, the contraction of the biceps results in movement of the forearm. The hand, which is attached to the forearm, also moves, indirectly, rather than directly.

For direct application, the resistance must be applied to the actual body part that is attached to and directly moved by contraction of the muscle you're trying to work. In a curl, this means that the resistance would have to be applied against the forearm instead of the hand.

In an actual curl, though, such direct application of resistance is of little importance. The relative strength of the

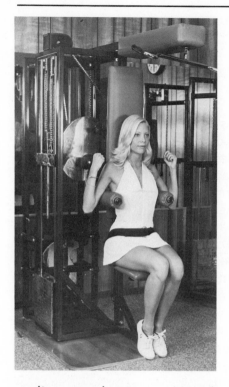

The latissimus dorsi muscles move the upper arms from an overhead position down and around the shoulder joints. To provide direct resistance for these large muscles, the resistance must be placed on the backs of the upper arms. The Nautilus behind neck machine provides direct resistance for the latissimus dorsi muscles.

curling muscles is not out of proportion to the strength of the forearm muscles involved in keeping the hand straight in line with the forearm during a curl. So in this case, other muscles do not limit your curling ability, even though the resistance is not directly applied.

In most exercises, the resistance must be applied directly in order to overcome the limitation of other, weaker muscles. Exercises designed for the large muscles of the torso suffer badly from indirect application of the resistance. Since the muscles of the arms are also involved in these exercises, the exertion must end when the arm muscles are exhausted. This exhaustion occurs long before the larger, stronger muscles of the torso have been worked heavily enough for best results.

Chinning-type exercises, for instance, are performed primarily for the purposes of working the larger muscles of the upper torso. But these exercises also involve the bending muscles of the arms. As a consequence, the relatively low strength of the arm muscles results in poor exercise for the torso muscles. Your exhausted arms force you to stop the exercise before your torso muscles have been properly worked.

To work the torso muscles correctly, the resistance must be applied directly to the body part that is actually attached to and moved by the muscles of the torso. In practice, the resistance must be directly applied against the upper arms. What happens to the forearms and hands during the exercise is not important so long, at least, as the forearms and hands do not get in the way of the movement. And in a Nautilus pullover machine, the resistance is applied directly against your upper arms. The large muscles of the torso can be worked directly without the limitations imposed by smaller and weaker muscles.

Most barbell exercises and most barbell-like exercises performed on a Universal machine do not provide such direct resistance. Isokinetic exercises, in general, suffer from the same limitations. There are a few exceptions in all these machines; a curl is a direct exercise regardless of how it is performed, a wrist curl is a direct exercise, and so are leg extensions and leg curls. But in general, direct exercise is provided only by Nautilus equipment.

RESISTANCE IN THE POSITION OF FULL-MUSCULAR CONTRACTION

Full-muscular contraction occurs in a position where additional movement is impossible. Obviously, an isokinetic form of exercise provides no work in the finishing position of an exercise. Isokinetic exercises provide resistance from friction, and friction is produced by movement. When movement stops, friction stops. Without friction there is no resistance, and without resistance there is no exercise. In isokinetic exercise there is no back pressure of negative work pulling against the muscles and therefore, no exercise in the finishing position of full-muscular contraction.

Neither do most barbell exercises or most Universal machine exercises provide work in the finishing position. In most of these exercises, the body parts are locked out under the resistance and the weight is supported entirely by the bones. Such lock-outs occur during all major barbell exercises and all major Universal machine exercises such as curls, all forms of pressing, squats, leg presses, and many other exercises. In these exercises, there is no effective resistance at the end of the movement. The lever arm of the resistance is reduced to zero, and no resistance is being applied to the muscles.

But there are exceptions. A few minor barbell exercises and Universal machine exercises do provide resistance in the finishing position. Some such exceptions are wrist curls, calf raises, and shoulder shrugs.

UNRESTRICTED SPEED OF MOVEMENT

In exercise, the speed of movement should not be limited. But since this is the basis of isokinetic forms of exercise, they suffer badly.

At the start of an isokinetic form of exercise, there is no resistance until the person's speed of movement reaches the pre-set speed of movement on the machine. There is obviously no resistance at the start of the isokinetic movement. And at the end of an isokinetic exercise, where any speed of movement is impossible, there is again no resistance. Isokinetic exercises are based on friction which results in limiting the speed of movement. This can be done by the use of an inertia-reel, a hydraulic cylinder, and perhaps in a few more ways, but the result is much the same no matter how accomplished.

The actual speed of movement during a properly performed exercise should vary during the exercise. During the first few repetitions the speed should be fairly slow and constant, without jerking. During later repetitions, as the muscles become tired, the speed should be slightly faster, but jerking must still be avoided. Finally, as the muscles reach a point of momentary exhaustion, the speed of movement is very slow.

The speed of movement in barbell exercises and in Universal machine exercises is not limited, so these exercises do not suffer from this limitation. Neither is the speed of movement limited in Nautilus exercises.

THE SUPERIORITY OF NAUTILUS

Ridiculous claims are being widely advertised for a number of forms of exercise. Almost all such exercises are supposedly full-range. But once you understand the facts, you can see these false claims in proper perspective. If an exercise is lacking any one of the 10 basic requirements, it cannot be a full-range exercise, no matter what the claims of uninformed promoters.

Most barbell and many machine exercises provide only four of the 10 requirements: positive work, negative work, pre-stretching, and unrestricted speed of movement. Isokinetic exercise machines generally provide only one of the basic requirements: positive work. But Nautilus single-joint rotary machines provide all 10 requirements.

When the requirements for full-range exercise are understood and applied in a practical fashion, it becomes possible to provide a form of exercise that involves all of a muscular structure. Only Nautilus machines make it possible to involve all of a muscular structure: the related body parts, the joints, the connective tissue, and even the bones. Such total exercise is capable of producing a level of strength and fitness that cannot be duplicated in any other fashion. Nautilus is the only form of exercise that is tailored to the requirements and the limitations of the body itself.

Remember, only Nautilus machines fulfill the requirements of full-range exercise.

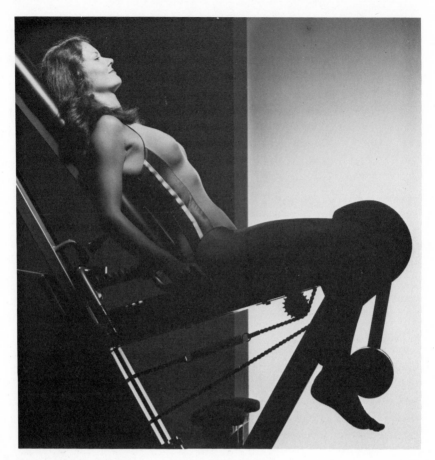

Leg extension machine.

nautilus training principles

While Nautilus equipment makes it possible to benefit dramatically from exercise, it does not offer easy results. Full-range exercise performed on Nautilus machines is demanding. It is by far the hardest recognized form of exercise. It happens fast, and it's enormously productive. But it was never intended to be easy.

Arthur Jones developed the hardest possible form of exertion by involving maximum possible muscle fibers in each exercise movement. If you want fast results, rest assured that properly performed Nautilus machine exercises will produce them more quickly than any other equipment. This statement sounds bold, but it's scientifically true.

A clear understanding of the following principles will assure you the best possible results from Nautilus machines.

INTENSITY

The building of strength is proportionate to the intensity of exercise. The higher the intensity, the better the muscles are stimulated. Performing a Nautilus exercise to the point of momentary muscular failure assures that you've trained to maximum intensity. Muscular failure means that no additional repetitions are possible. It is only by working to this extent that you engage a maximum number of muscle fibers.

The first few repetitions on a Nautilus machine are merely preparation, doing little to increase strength. These repetitions are of limited value because the intensity is low. The final repetitions are productive because the intensity is high.

Many people refuse to perform these last several repetitions. But those forced repetitions are the most effective. A Nautilus exercise should not be considered completed until you just can't perform another repetition in correct form.

PROGRESSION

The cornerstone of Nautilus training is progression. Progression means attempting to increase the work load every training session. With each workout, you should try to add another repetition, additional resistance, or both. Experience has shown that at least 8 repetitions should be performed and not more than 12. If you cannot achieve 8 repetitions, the resistance is too heavy. If you can perform more than 12 repetitions, it is too light. When you can perform 12 repetitions or more, it is the signal to increase the resistance on that Nautilus machine by approximately 5 percent at the next workout.

Nautilus machines are made with 10-pound weight increments. The percentage of increase can be reduced if you simply pin a small 1¼-, 2½-, or 5-pound barbell plate to the weight stack. By using small weight increments such as these, you can progress in a more systematic manner.

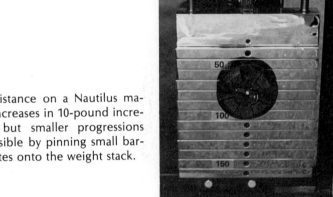

The resistance on a Nautilus machine increases in 10-pound increments, but smaller progressions are possible by pinning small barbell plates onto the weight stack.

FORM

The style of performance is very important if maximum benefit is to be obtained from a Nautilus training program. Proper form includes both speed and range of movement.

Repetitions performed in a slow, smooth manner apply steady force through the entire movement. Fast repetitions apply force to only a small portion at the beginning and the end of the movement. When a resistance is jerked or thrown, three or four times the actual force required to move the resistance is directed to the joints and muscles. This is both ineffective and dangerous.

The range of movement of each repetition, from full extension to full flexion, should be as great as possible. To contract at all, a muscle must produce movement. To contract fully, however, a muscle must produce a full range of movement. If the movement resulting from muscular contraction is less than full range, the entire length of the muscle is not involved in the work. Improved performance and prevention of injury are most likely when the muscles have been strengthened in every position over a full range of possible movement.

ACCENTUATE THE NEGATIVE

For best results, each repetition should be performed in a negative-emphasized manner. The performance of Nautilus exercise requires the raising and lowering of resistance. When you raise the weight stack, you're moving against the resistance of gravity and performing positive work. Lowering a weight under control brings gravity into play in another fashion. The lowering portion of an exercise is termed negative work.

In a Nautilus biceps curl, you perform both positive and negative work during each repetition. Positive resistance is involved when the arms are bending and raising the weight. When the arms are straightening and lowering the weight, that is negative resistance. Up is positive; down is negative. This is true for each Nautilus machine.

Dr. Paavo Komi of Finland and other physiologists have recently determined that for strength-building purposes, the negative part of an exercise has much more value than the positive portion. Nautilus machines are more productive when ways are devised to accentuate the negative part of each movement.

In normal positive-negative exercise performed on Nautilus equipment, you should always concentrate on the lowering part of the movement. If it takes two seconds to lift a weight smoothly, it should take about four seconds to lower it.

To perform negative-only exercise, you need to select a heavier weight than you would use normally. Initially, you should use about 40 percent more weight than you can handle for 10 repetitions in a normal positive-negative manner. With this additional amount of weight on the Nautilus machine, you have one or two assistants, or instructors, lift the movement arm to the contracted position. It is then your job to lower the resistance back to the starting position.

During the first two or three repetitions, it should take approximately 8 to 10 seconds per repetition to lower the resistance in a slow, even manner. It should be possible for you to stop and reverse the movement of these repetitions, although no attempt should be made to do so.

If the weight has been correctly selected, the middle three or four repetitions should be performed slightly faster, approximately 4 to 5 seconds per repetition. In these repetitions, you should be able to stop the movement, but no longer able to reverse it.

During the last repetition, it becomes impossible to stop the downward movement, even though you can control it. The exercise is finally terminated when the downward movement can no longer be controlled.

Properly performed, negative-only exercise is a very effective style of Nautilus training. But there are problems, since it is usually necessary to have someone lift the movement arm for you.

A few exercises can be performed in a negative-only manner without help. Negative chins and dips on the multi-exercise machine can be done by climbing into the top position with the legs and slowly lowering with the arms. Thus, your lower body is doing the positive work and your upper body is doing the negative work. This style of training can also be performed on at least four Nautilus machines, called Omni. In most cases, a foot-pedal attachment allows you to leg-press the movement arm into the contracted position and lower the resistance with your upper body. But since your upper body is weaker than your lower body, you cannot work your lower body in this fashion. That is why negative-accentuated training was invented.

Negative-accentuated training does not require helpers. Nor does it require anywhere near as much resistance as negative-only training. You can use Nautilus machines that have single connected movement arms.

The leg extension machine offers a good example of negative-accentuated exercise. If you can handle 100 pounds for 10 repetitions in a normal manner, you should use 70 pounds here—in other words, 70 percent of the weight you normally handle.

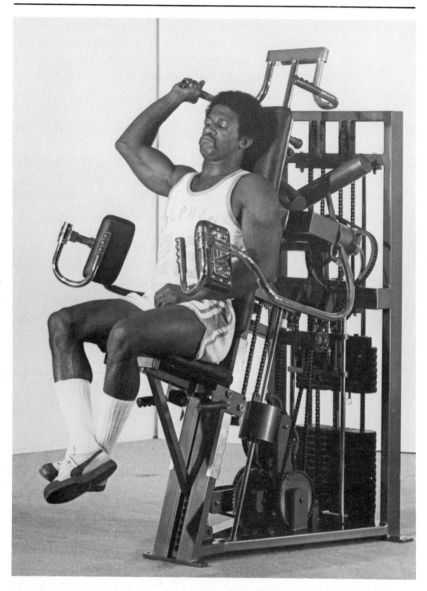

The lowering phase of each machine should always be emphasized. To perform negative-accentuated overhead presses on the Nautilus double shoulder machine, the trainee should lift the resistance with both arms and lower it slowly with one arm, then lift the resistance again with two arms and lower it with the other arm.

The movement arm should be lifted with both legs. Pause in the contracted position, and smoothly transfer the resistance from both legs to the right leg. Then, slowly lower the resistance in about 8 seconds, using only the right leg. Lift it back to the top position with both legs, pause, and lower this time with the left leg, again in a slow, even manner. Up with two, down with one, up with two again, down with the other. This should continue until you can no longer raise the weight to the contracted position.

If the weight is selected correctly, you should reach a point of momentary failure about the eleventh or twelfth lifting repetition. When you can perform 12 repetitions, increase the resistance 5 percent. A properly performed set of negative-accentuated exercise should consist of 8 to 12 lifting movements, plus 4 to 6 negative movements performed by the right leg and an equal number by the left.

Other negative-accentuated exercises that can be performed on various machines are the leg curl, leg press, calf raise, hip and back extension, pullover, overhead press, decline press, biceps curl, and triceps extension.

DURATION

If each Nautilus exercise is done properly in a high-intensity fashion, brief workouts must be the rule. High-intensity exercise has an effect on the entire system that can be either good or bad; low-intensity work has almost no effect at all. If high-intensity work is followed by an adequate period of rest, muscular growth and increase in strength will result. Intensive work, however, must not be overdone.

Many athletes mistakenly perform too much exercise. They do too many different movements, too many sets, and too many workouts within a given period of time. When an excess amount of Nautilus exercise is performed, total recovery between workouts becomes impossible. So does high-intensity training.

You can perform brief and infrequent high-intensity exercise, or long and frequent low-intensity workouts. But you cannot perform long and frequent Nautilus exercise involving a high intensity of work. That will only result in large-scale losses in both muscular mass and strength. It can also result in total exhaustion.

Understanding the requirements for a productive style of high-intensity exercise allows selection of the best exercises for a particular purpose. In most cases, not more than 12 different Nautilus exercises should be performed in any one workout. The lower body should have 4–6 exercises and the upper body 6–8. If you push or are pushed to the supreme effort in each of 12 exercises, you will not be able to perform more than one set.

A set of 10 repetitions performed in proper style should take about one minute to complete. Allowing one minute between exercises, most athletes should be able to complete 12 Nautilus exercises in less than 25 minutes. As you work yourself into better condition, the time between exercises should be reduced. It is entirely possible to go through an entire workout of 12 Nautilus exercises in less than 15 minutes. Such a workout not only develops muscular size and strength, but also develops a high level of cardiovascular endurance.

MORE IS NOT BETTER

An advanced trainee does not need more Nautilus exercise than a beginner; rather, the need changes in the direction of "harder but less."

Beginning trainees usually show acceptable strength gains on most types of exercise programs, even though they may perform several sets of more than 12 repetitions in each training session. They are able to make this progress, at least for a while, because they are not strong enough to use up all their recovery ability. As they get stronger, however, they do use that recovery ability, and their progress stops. The stronger the individual becomes, the greater resistance he handles and the greater inroads he makes into his recovery ability. So the advanced trainee must reduce his overall Nautilus exercises from 12 to 10, and train only at high intensity twice a week. On Monday, he might train hard, on Wednesday less strenuously, and on Friday hard again. The Wednesday workout would not stimulate growth, but it would keep his muscles from atrophying. It would permit growth by not making significant inroads into the athlete's recovery ability.

ORDER

Workouts should begin with the largest muscle groups and proceed downward to the smallest. This is important for two reasons: working the largest muscles first causes the greatest degree of overall body stimulation; and it is impossible to reach momentary muscular exhaustion in a large muscle if the smaller muscle group serving as a link between the resistance and the large muscle groups have been previously exhausted. Thus it is important to work the largest muscles first while the system is still capable of working with the desired intensity.

For best results, the order of exercise should be as follows:

1. Hips and lower back
2. Legs
   a. Quadriceps
   b. Hamstrings
   c. Calves
3. Torso
   a. Back
   b. Shoulders
   c. Chest
4. Arms
   a. Triceps
   b. Biceps
   c. Forearms
5. Neck

VARIETY

The human body quickly grows accustomed to almost any kind of activity. Once this happens, no amount of participation in the same activity will provide growth stimulation. It is therefore important to provide many forms of variation in Nautilus training. Variation can be made in several different ways. Weight or repetitions can be varied for each workout. The exercises can be changed occasionally, alternated, or performed in a different sequence. And training days can be varied.

FREQUENCY

You should rest at least 48 hours, but not more than 96 hours, between Nautilus workouts.

High-intensity Nautilus exercise causes a complex chemical reaction inside a muscle. If given time, the muscle will compensate by causing certain cells to get bigger and stronger. High-intensity exercise is, therefore, necessary to stimulate muscular growth. But it is not the only requirement. The stimulated muscle must be given time to grow.

Research performed at Ohio State University by Drs. Edward Fox and Robert Bartels has shown that there should be approximately 48 hours between workouts, but 72 to 96 hours between sessions are required for extremely strong athletes. High levels of muscular size and strength begin to decrease and atrophy after 96 hours of normal activity. This means that you should exercise every other day.

An every-other-day, three times per week Nautilus program also seems to provide the body with the needed irregularity of training. A first workout is performed on Monday. Two days later, a second workout is performed on Wednesday, and a third on Friday. Thus, on Sunday, the system is expecting and is prepared for a fourth workout, but it does not come. Instead, it comes a day later, on the next Monday when the body is neither expecting nor prepared for it. This schedule of training prevents the body from falling into a regular routine. Since the system is never quite able to adjust to this irregularity of training, growth is stimulated.

SUPERVISION

Perhaps an individual can push himself to a 100-percent effort occasionally, or on two or three Nautilus exercises, but experience proves that this is virtually impossible to do consistently.

Nautilus high-intensity exercise is not easy. Properly performed, it is very demanding, and it is not surprising that few people can do it on their own initiative. An instructor is needed to supervise and urge most trainees to work at the required level of intensity.

An example from running should help clarify this concept:

An athlete can run a quarter mile in 50 seconds. When he runs this, it is a 100-percent effort. His pain during the last 100 yards will be almost unbearable. He rationalizes, therefore, that if he slows slightly to run the distance in 55 seconds, he will probably get 90-percent results. If he repeats the 55-second quarter three times, he falsely reasons, he will accomplish more than by running the track one time with 100-percent effort.

But he will never get the degree of results from running 55-second quarters three times that he would have by running the track with one 100-percent effort. It is the 100-percent effort that forces his body to over-compensate and get stronger. Ninety-percent efforts, regardless of how many times they are repeated, will never approach the results attained by one 100-percent effort.

The same applies to building strength. If you can do 11 repetitions in a stringent effort on a given Nautilus exercise, but instead stop at 10, you have not reached your potential.

This is why supervision is all-important. You cannot push yourself hard enough. You need a supervisor to tell you when to slow down, to hold your head back, and relax your lower body when working your upper body. You must be reminded to eliminate excessive gripping and facial expressions, to do the last repetition of each exercise, and to perform numerous other activities that make each Nautilus exercise harder and more productive.

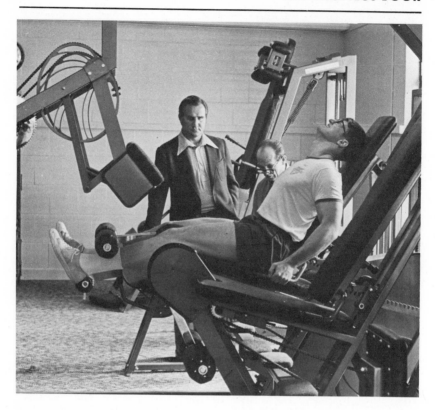

For best results, Nautilus training should be closely supervised. Here, Arthur Jones supervises an athlete performing leg extensions, as Don Shula observes.

KEEPING ACCURATE RECORDS

You should keep accurate records of workout-by-workout progress. This can be done on a card that lists the exercises with ample space to the right for recording the date, resistance, repetitions, and training time.

WARMING UP

Warming up may be, as some authorities believe, more psychological than physiological. But there is ample evidence to support the case for warming up as a safeguard against injury. On the warm-up, the cartilages of the knee increase their thickness and provide a better fit of the surfaces of the knee joint. Friction-like resistance of the muscle cells is reduced by the higher temperature of the body, and the elasticity of the tendons and ligaments is increased. The change to higher temperature not only augments speed of movement and power potential, but minimizes risk of injury.

A few degrees' rise in temperature of the muscle cells speeds up the production of energy by one-third. These changes in the human mechanism are similar to those that occur in an automobile as it warms up.

Almost any sequence of light calisthenic movements can be used as a general warm-up to precede a vigorous Nautilus training session. Suggested movements include head rotation, side bend, trunk twist, squat, and stationary cycling. A minute or so of each movement will be sufficient. Specific warming up for each body part occurs during the first four repetitions of each Nautilus exercise.

NAUTILUS TRAINING FOR WOMEN

Most women firmly believe that if they participate in Nautilus exercise, their muscles will become large and unfeminine in appearance. But the truth is that it is virtually impossible for a woman to develop large muscles. The larger, more defined muscle mass in men is no accident. It is the direct effect of the male hormone testosterone upon the growth mechanism of the male's body. Before puberty, there is little difference between the muscular size and strength of boys and girls. Once puberty begins, testosterone from the male testes and estrogen from female ovaries enter the bloodstream, triggering the development of the appropriate secondary sexual characteristics.

A small percentage of women do have large muscles, particularly in their legs, which in most cases may be inherited or the result of an above-average amount of testosterone in the system. The adrenal glands and the sex glands in both men and women secrete a small amount of the nondominant hormone. If a larger than usual amount of testosterone is secreted in a female, she has the potential for greater muscle development. There are also men who have an above-average amount of estrogen in their systems which tends to give them a feminine-like appearance.

Generally speaking, 99.99 percent of American women could not develop large muscles under any circumstances. But Nautilus exercise is worthwhile because it strengthens and conditions their muscles and prevents injuries.

12 RULES FOR NAUTILUS TRAINING

1. Perform one set of 4–6 exercises for the lower body and 6–8 exercises for the upper body, and no more than 12 exercises in any workout.

2. Select a resistance on each exercise that allows you to do between 8–12 repetitions.

3. Continue each exercise until no additional repetitions

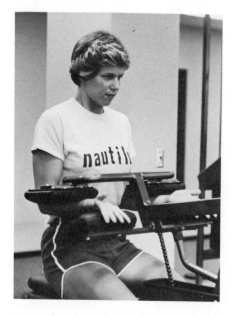

Because they have long ne-glected their muscular strength, women may have more to gain from Nautilus training than men.

are possible. When 12 or more repetitions are performed, increase the resistance by approximately 5 percent at the next workout.

4. Work the largest muscles first and move quickly from one exercise to the next. This procedure develops cardiovascular endurance.

5. Concentrate on flexibility by slowly stretching during the first three repetitions of each exercise.

6. Accentuate the lowering portion of each repetition.

7. Move slower, never faster, if in doubt about the speed of movement.

8. Do everything possible to isolate and work each large muscle group to exhaustion.

9. Attempt constantly to increase the number of repetitions or the amount of weight, or both. But do not sacrifice form in an attempt to produce results.

10. Train no more than three times a week.

11. Keep accurate records—date, resistance, repetitions, and overall training time—of each workout.

12. Vary the workouts often.

WORDS OF CAUTION

Before beginning a Nautilus training program, you should undergo a medical examination. Vigorous exercise can be dangerous to some people. Intense physical activity coupled with certain environmental conditions may aggravate existing asthmatic conditions. People with a tendency toward high blood pressure should be closely supervised in any heavy lifting or straining exercises that may cause temporary increases in that pressure. Those over the age of 35, and coronary-prone younger people who possess high-risk factors, should obtain a stress-test electrocardiogram. Stress tests are particularly important to those who have the following risk factors: overweight, hypertension, diabetes, sedentary life style, cigarette smoking, and a family history of early heart disease.

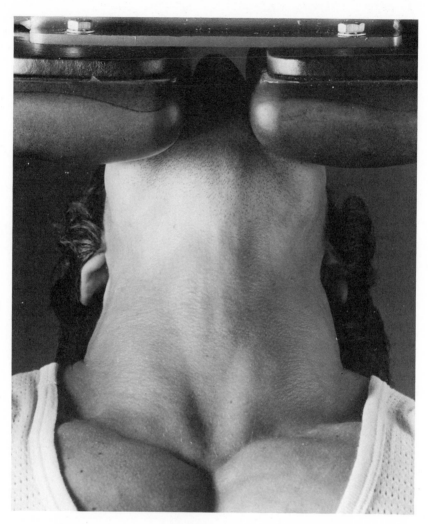

4-way neck machine

CHAPTER THREE

heredity and training

Inherited characteristics play a dominating role in every individual's life. These inherited characteristics are transmitted from generation to generation by a complex system of genes. The study of genes is called genetics.

"How one thinks," Arthur Jones says, "is determined by genetics." Not only is mental capacity determined by genetics, but physical potential such as height, bodily proportions, fat, muscle mass, and other attributes come to us from our progenitors. Obviously, then, great athletes, like musicians, poets, actors, and painters are largely born, not made.

O.J. Simpson would have never become a football superstar without somebody fleet of foot in his ancestry.

Wilt Chamberlain is certainly not the only seven-foot-tall man in the world. But his bodily proportions, neurological efficiency, skeletal formation, lack of body fat, and muscle length combine with above-average intelligence to make him the greatest basketball scorer in history.

Entirely different genes made Nadia Comaneci, at five foot and 87 pounds, the greatest female gymnast the world has ever seen.

All three of these famous athletes could have never attained pre-eminence in their special field without their inherited characteristics. But these inherited traits would have never matured without the right conditioning and coaching.

Nautilus machines are capable of furnishing correct conditioning for any athlete in any sport. But it can produce results only within the limits of the individual's inherited capabilities. Nautilus cannot make plain Jane into a champion gymnast any more than it can make John Doe a professional basketball star.

GENETIC FACTORS

Bodily Proportions

Superior athletes have bodily proportions ideally suited to their particular sport. Dick Butkus had ideal proportions for a football middle linebacker: long torso, short legs, wide hips, narrow shoulders, and long arms. Jesse Owens had a short torso, narrow hips, long legs, and a favorable ratio of the lower to the upper leg, all of which gave him the potential to become a very fast sprinter.

Olga Korbut, former world champion gymnast, had small proportions which enabled her to perform skillfully under limited conditions. Maren Seidler, the women's national shot put champion, has large proportions that perfectly fit her sport. The bodily proportions essential to Olga would be disastrous to Maren.

From a mechanical point of view, there are bodily proportions especially suited to each sport. Coaches and athletes need to be conscious of such inherited anatomical traits. Appropriate height, torso length, shoulder width, length of arms, leg length, and the ratio of the lower to the upper leg

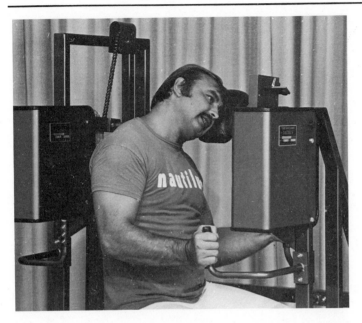

Dick Butkus, shown on the Nautilus 4-way neck machine, had the ideal combination of genetic factors for a middle linebacker.

are crucial determinants of an individual's ability to perform.

These widths and lengths, the various attachments of tendons to bone, and the strength and musculature of the body form its levers of locomotion. These size relationships are part of the field of physiology called biomechanics.

Skeletal Formation

Skeletal formation determines bodily proportions. An athlete must possess bones large enough to support heavy musculature. But his bones must not exceed a certain size, or he may lose the necessary aesthetic qualities contingent upon bone structure. The aspiring athlete with the fragile bone structure of Woody Allen could hardly hope to develop the heavy-duty muscles of Lou Ferrigno. Neither can an individual with the gargantuan skeleton of Paul Anderson ever develop the sweeping symmetry of Steve Reeves. Once a person's bones pass a certain size, the joints tend to become so thick that the taper of a muscle belly cannot fit into a small tight joint.

Neurological Efficiency

Neurological efficiency, as it applies to physical fitness, is the relationship between the nervous system and the muscles. The brain activates the muscles required for each movement, and determines the amount of muscle power from the available supply of usable resources. People with high levels of neurological efficiency are able to contract greater percentages of their muscle masses. This places athletes with lower usable levels at a disadvantage.

Recent research undertaken in Canada reveals that neurological efficiency varies greatly among people. Most people were found to be able to contract, in an utmost effort, about 30 percent of a tested muscle group. A few individuals managed 40 percent. Their muscles were no better or worse than others. They merely had the ability to contract a greater percentage of muscle fibers. At the lower end of the normal curve is the 10-percent athlete. Occasionally there is a 50-percent individual in neurological efficiency. But for every 50-percenter, there is also a 10-percenter. Both these extremes are rare. A 50-percent individual would be a genetic freak in strength. A 10-percent person would be a "motor moron," hardly able to walk in a straight line.

These are proportional figures, but an under-achieving 50-percent athlete can be beaten by a 30-percent competitor functioning neurologically at his best. The 50-percent athlete may be so accustomed to coasting that he has never learned to make a vigorous effort during training or competition. This is a major paradox limiting athletic performance. Being able to assess the potential of a player in these terms provides the coach with the knowledge of what he can expect from each member of the team. The 50-percent athlete cannot hide his potential with average performances, nor can the genetically average athlete defeat the gifted athlete with the will to work.

Muscle Length

The *length* of an individual's muscles is the most important factor in determining the potential size of those muscles. The longer a person's muscles, the greater the cross-sectional area and the volume of his muscles can become.

The most easily measured muscle lengths are the triceps of the arms, the gastrocnemious of the calves, and the flexors of the forearms. If two men flex the long head of the triceps, with the arm down by the side, and measure the length of this muscle, vastly different measurements could result. The length of the first man's triceps might measure 6 inches, while the second man's might be 9. The length of the second man's triceps would therefore be 50 percent greater than the first man's. Consequently, the second man has the potential of 2.25 times as much cross-sectional area $(1.5 \times 1.5 = 2.25)$ and 3.375 as much volume or mass

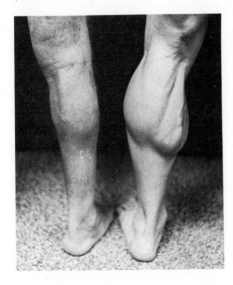

This photograph shows the difference between short and long muscles and their effect on the mass of the calf. The man on the right has greater size to his calf primarily because of his long gastrocnemius and soleus muscles.

(1.5 × 1.5 × 1.5 = 3.375) to his triceps. Untrained, both these men might have approximately the same arm size, but with proper training, the second man can have a much stronger and larger muscle.

Just because a person has a short triceps does not mean that all his muscles are short. Differences are even observed from one side of the body to the other, and from body part to body part. It is the rare individual who has uniform potential over the entire body. Often we see the body builder who has great arms and legs but suffers a noticeable deficiency in the torso. Or there is the athlete with large thighs and small calves; this is most prevalent among blacks. Most blacks inherit short gastrocnemious muscles and long tendons in their lower legs.

Body Fat

All people are born with adipose cells which specialize in accumulating fat. Many nutritional authorities think that the number of these cells is genetically predetermined. According to these authorities, family fat deposits are inherited in the same way as height, coloring, nose shapes, and muscle length.

Researchers have found that the average non-obese person has about 25 to 30 billion fat cells throughout his body. For the moderately obese, the number of fat cells is about 50 billion. For the extremely obese, the number of fat cells may be as high as 237 billion. Perhaps this explains why some people think they were destined to be fat, or find it very difficult to lose fat permanently.

During the first year of life, cell numbers increase fairly rapidly. The total number of fat cells is about three times greater at one year of age than at birth. Scientists believe that most fat cells existing prior to birth are formed during the last three months of pregnancy. After the first year of life, cell numbers increase more gradually, to the age of about 10. The number of fat cells formed continues to increase after the age of 13, and during the growth spurt of adolescence until adulthood, at which time there is little, if any, further increase in the number of fat cells.

Thus there appear to be three critical periods when the number of fat cells significantly increases. The first period is during the last trimester of pregnancy, the second is during the first year of life, and the third occurs during the adolescent growth spurt.

It is during adulthood that the total number of fat cells cannot be altered. It should be pointed out, however, that there is still no substantial data to indicate clearly that the final number of adult fat cells cannot be modified through some form of intervention at an earlier period of life. If fat cells can be altered, it is likely to be accomplished by a combination of two factors: modification of early nutrition and proper exercise.

Somatotypes

Research on various body types has been done by numerous authorities. Foremost of these is Dr. W.H. Sheldon, an American scholar, who categorized human beings by a system called somatotyping. Dr. Sheldon concluded that all the infinite variety of body types could be analyzed according to three tendencies. An individual's body could be classified by analyzing to what degree each of these three variables was represented.

He named the three variables endomorphy, mesomorphy, and ectomorphy. *Endomorphy* is the tendency to soft roundness in the body. *Mesomorphy* is the tendency to muscularity. *Ectomorphy* is the tendency toward slimness.

The basic endomorph is stocky with a large round body, a short thick neck, and short arms and legs with fatter upper arms and thighs.

The perfect mesomorph is strongly built with broad muscular shoulders and chest, very muscular arms and legs, and

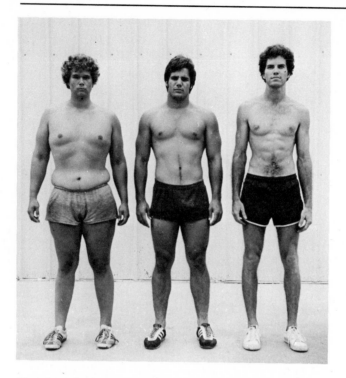

The three basic somatotypes are shown above. *Left to right:* endomorphy, mesomorphy, and ectomorphy.

little body fat. (Other body types can develop larger muscles, but not to the same degree as a mesomorph.)

The prototype ectomorph is tall and thin with a narrow body, thin arms and legs, little body fat, and stringy muscles.

Dr. Sheldon drew a scale for each variable of body type. An individual could be scored from 1 to 7 on each tendency. But if the score was high on one, it could not be high on others. By listing all three scores, the person's body type was recorded and analyzed, and somatotyped.

An extreme endomorph would be 7-1-1, an extreme mesomorph 1-7-1, and an extreme ectomorph 1-1-7. In reality, such extremes seldom occur, but neither are most people an average 4-4-4.

Dr. Sheldon's system assumes that the somatotype does not change with age, diet, or exercise. But some experts believe that somatotype can be partially altered by exercise during puberty. All agree, however, that by age 16 or 17, everybody's basic type has been permanently established.

A knowledge of which sport favors which somatotype can guide a young athlete in deciding athletic pursuits. Somatotyping an athlete is done by analyzing three photographs using carefully standardized postures. The scoring is a matter of judgment, but experienced assessors rate the same body very similarly.

INTELLIGENT TRAINING

Bodily proportions, skeletal formation, neurological efficiency, muscle length, and body fat are all genetic traits that cannot be changed by training. Only training, however, can activate them to capacity. True, genetic qualities are limiting factors. But this is not to say that a given individual cannot improve his existing development, performance, or appearance. With strict attention to training methods, eating habits, and coaching, every person could reach the upper limits of his particular genetic potential.

Even the chosen few who are born with almost perfect combinations of genetic factors necessary for success in a given activity will improve faster if they approach their training intelligently. An aspiring champion, whose ultimate potential may be less than that of a mesomorphic opponent, may still achieve greater success by the use of applied intelligence. The ultimate, however, occurs when superior genetic factors are married to the intellectual capacity to utilize them. This combination cannot be beaten. Genetic factors exist and generally cannot be altered.

The following concepts summarize the importance of genetics and Nautilus training:

1. From a biomechanical point of view, there are certain bodily proportions and bone structures that are necessary

for success in building strength and demonstrating strength. There are also ideal bodily proportions for success in a given sport.

2. Individuals with high levels of neurological efficiency get faster results from Nautilus training. These people also have a marked advantage in competition where great muscular strength is required.

3. The mesomorphic individual has greater probability of success in Nautilus training than does the endomorphic or ectomorphic individual.

4. The length of a given muscle determines its ultimate size potential. Any athlete desiring large muscle size must be blessed with longer than average muscle bellies.

5. Where an individual stores fat on his body, and to what degree, are genetically predetermined. Many bodybuilders who are trying to obtain great muscular definition fail to realize that this may be impossible. Great muscular definition not only requires that the individual have a low percentage of body fat, but that he store the majority of that fat on the inside of the body. Most people store the majority of their fat under the skin all over their bodies.

The superior athlete was born with the genetic possibility to be a great basketball player, tennis player, wrestler, runner, bodybuilder, or any other kind of sports performer. His training and coaching were important for his success, but not as important as his genetics.

An individual desiring to be taller might assume, after watching several professional basketball games, that bouncing a ball would make him taller. After trying various ball-bouncing routines with no success, he might conclude that bouncing a ball has no effect on his height. He might also realize that if an individual has the genetic potential to be taller, he will grow taller whether he bounces the ball or not. If he grew in height, it would be his genetic inheritance and not his ball bouncing.

To play professional basketball, an individual generally has to be very tall. He has to learn the skills of basketball at a young age. This is not to say, however, that all people cannot learn the skills of basketball and enjoy playing the game. But there is little probability of an individual's playing professional basketball unless he has inherited genes that make him tall.

To win the Mr. America Contest or other bodybuilding championships, an individual must first have the genetic potential. He must have the ideal bodily proportions and bone structure, long muscle bellies in the appropriate places, and the ability to store fat deep inside of the body rather than between the skin and the muscles.

Proper Nautilus training will not make a man into a Mr. America unless he has the genetic potential. Few people have that potential. But proper Nautilus training will vastly improve anyone's muscular size, strength, shape, and condition, and will do this quickly. It will not, however, make a mediocre athlete into a world champion. Champions are largely born, not made.

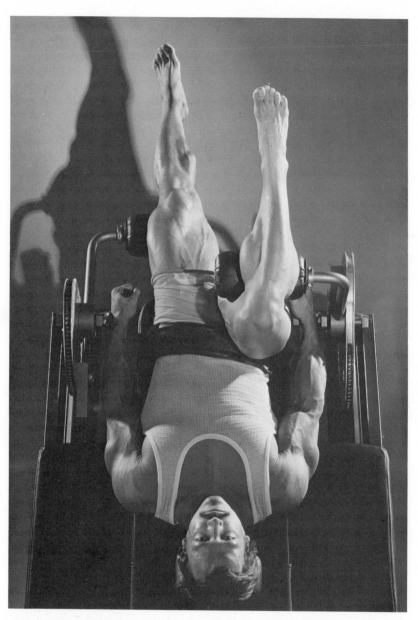

Hip and back machine

CHAPTER FOUR

hips and lower back

In Nautilus Fitness Centers across the country, people are mistakenly confusing the reduction of the hips with developing a big bottom. The hips and buttocks are among the most misunderstood parts of the human body.

Should the size of these muscles be reduced or increased?

Should women exercise the buttocks in a fashion different from men?

Is sitting the primary purpose of the buttocks?

The answer to these questions comes from an understanding of the human anatomy.

FUNCTION OF THE BUTTOCKS

The buttocks are used for sitting, since their covering is a thick layer of fatty tissue which acts as a natural cushion. The primary function of the buttocks, however, is not sitting, but the forceful extension of the hip. This forceful extension of

47

the hip is controlled by the largest and strongest muscles of the body, the gluteus maximus. All running, jumping, squatting, and intensive pushing is made possible by the gluteus maximus muscles.

Anyone involved in running and jumping sports can improve his performance by strengthening the gluteal muscles. Women concerned about the appearance of the buttocks area can, by keeping the gluteus maximus muscles as strong as possible, create a dimple-free sleekness to the overlying skin. Those who are troubled by low-back pain, and at least 20 million Americans are, can add considerable support to the back and spinal column by keeping the buttocks in strong condition.

If by chance someone developed the muscles of the buttocks to a disproportionate degree, then lack of activity for several days would result in automatic atrophy of the unused muscles. Muscles that are increased in size and strength by exercise do not remain in that condition unless they are frequently taxed to their limits.

Women who are concerned with overly fat hips should understand that this has little to do with large gluteus maximus muscles. This state is usually the result of the inherited tendency in many women to store above average amounts of fat on the backsides of their bodies. If this is the case, and it will be with numerous women, the proper combination of diet and exercise can correct the condition. But it will not alter anyone's tendency to be disproportionately fat in the hips.

Women should train in the same way as men, using the same exercises, repetitions, and sets. A woman's muscles should be treated exactly the same as a man's.

NAUTILUS HIP AND BACK MACHINE

The Nautilus hip and back machine was one of the first pieces of exercise equipment that Arthur Jones designed. The early model consisted of a single movement arm, the resistance had to be supplied by barbell plates, and there was no get-in/get-out device. It took several strong people to pull the movement arm to the contracted position as the trainee positioned himself on the axes of rotation and buckled down.

Since 1970, there have been at least a dozen improvements of the original hip and back machine. The current model, called duosymmetric/polycontractile, is much safer than some of the earlier versions, and it offers even better results.

DUOSYMMETRIC/POLYCONTRACTILE HIP AND BACK

1. Enter machine from front by separating movement arms.

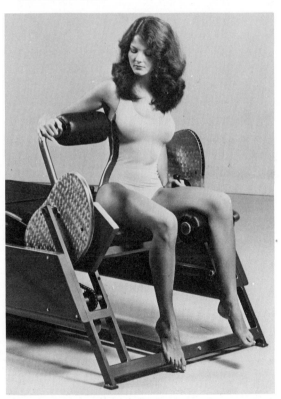

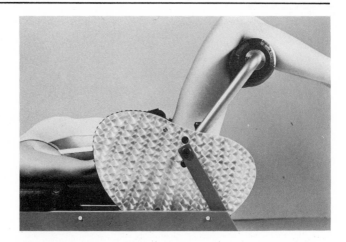

2. Lie on back with both legs over roller pads.
3. Align hip joints with axes of cams.

4. Fasten seat belt and grasp handles lightly.

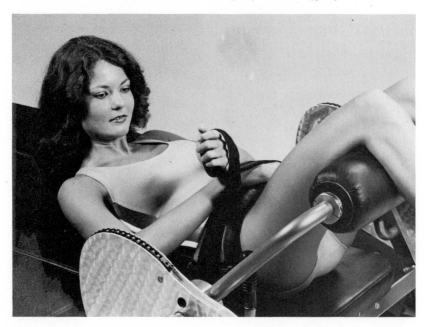

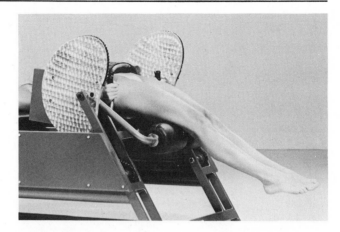

5. Extend both legs and at the same time push back with arms.

6. Keep one leg at full extension; allow other leg to bend and come back as far as possible.
7. Stretch.

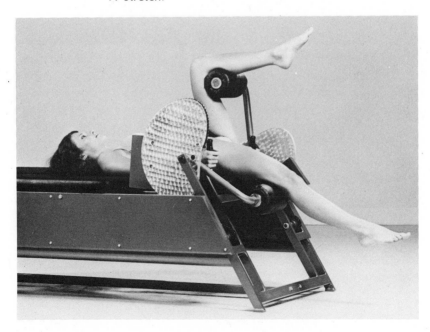

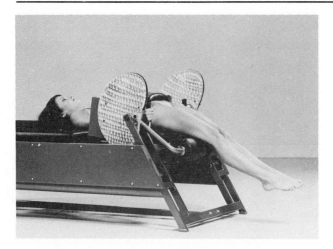

8. Push out until it joins other leg at extension.
9. Pause, arch lower back, and contract buttocks. In contracted position, keep legs straight, knees together, and toes pointed.
10. Repeat with other leg.

MULTI-EXERCISE MACHINE

Stiff-Legged Deadlift

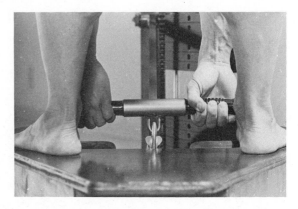

1. Move a 20-inch raised platform in position on the multi-exercise machine.
2. Attach the small handle to machine's movement arm.
3. Place feet on either side of platform.
4. Grasp handle with an under-and-over grip.

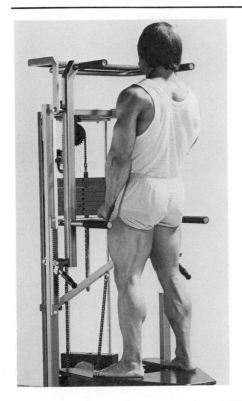

5. Lift movement arm to a standing position.

6. Keep knees locked and lower resistance to the stretched position.

7. Return to standing position and repeat.

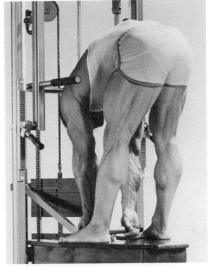

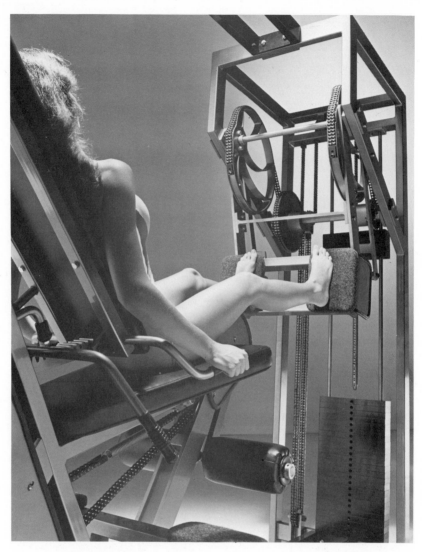

Compound leg machine

CHAPTER FIVE

legs

The leg is a marvelous structure. Long, lean, and shapely, a symmetrical pair can go a long way toward bringing their owner fame on the athletic field, recognition on the dance floor, or admiration on the beach.

The leg, unfortunately, is one of the most vulnerable parts of the body. Most everyone has suffered from ankle sprains. While ankle sprains are seldom permanently disabling, a knee injury can end an athlete's career as fast as he can say, "crackback block."

The knee is the largest and most complex joint of the body. A multiplicity of ligaments give the knee its stability. Crossing on top of the ligaments are the important muscles and tendons of the thigh and calf. There is no way to strengthen ligaments and tendons without working the muscles that connect to and surround them.

The muscles of the legs must be kept strong to protect the joints from injury. Strong legs not only prevent injuries, but improve performance in any running and jumping activity. Strong legs also contribute to overall fitness and body appearance.

KNEE AND THIGH

Although the knee is the largest joint in the body, from an architectural point of view, it is one of the weakest. Its structural weakness is due to the fact that in no position of flexion or extension are the bones ever in more than partial contact. This is especially important to the athlete because the knees support his weight, and stopping and starting movements put tremendous pressure on the knee joints.

The knee is essentially a hinge held together by a system of ligaments and tendons. There are 13 distinct ligaments that enter into its strength and support.

Of equal importance are a number of powerful muscles that cross the knee. The four muscles of the quadriceps and the three muscles of the hamstrings provide a tripod effect around the knee joint. Strong quadriceps and hamstring muscles offer the first line of defense against injury. The large muscles of the quadriceps and hamstrings also contribute to the size and strength of the thigh.

ANKLE AND CALF

In some ways the ankle joint functionally resembles the knee. Both joints bear most of the body's weight, allow motion predominately in the same direction, are supported by strong ligaments on either side, and are occasionally injured and later reinjured.

Bones and ligaments are the ankles' chief stability. Every aspect of the ankle is supported by a maze of ligaments and arranged to offer maximum support with maximum mobility. The strongest sets of ligaments are on the medial (inside) and lateral (outside) of the ankle. The ligaments restrict excess foot inversion and eversion. When the ligaments are damaged, so is the ability to maintain proper ankle stability, and recurrent sprains are a result.

Muscle tendons that cross the ankle on either side also aid in stabilization. On the medial side, the posterior tibial tendon offers ankle support, while on the lateral side the peroneal tendons exert their force.

The rounded form of the calf is primarily a result of the mass of two muscles, the gastrocnemius and soleus. These muscles insert into the heel bone by way of the Achilles tendon. They also cross the back of the knee joint. The gastroc-soleus muscles are the prime mover for ankle extension and they assist the hamstrings in knee flexion.

COMPOUND LEG MACHINE

Leg Extension

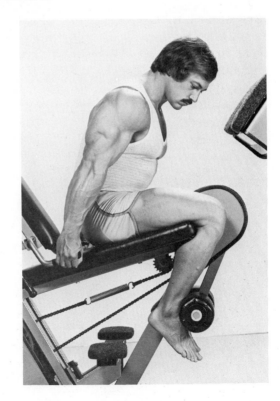

1. Place feet behind roller pads with knees snug against seat.
2. Adjust seat back to comfortable position.

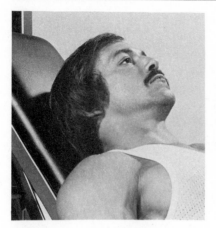 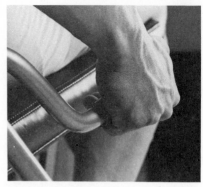

4. Grasp handles lightly.

3. Keep head and shoulders against seat back.

5. Straighten both legs smoothly.
6. Pause.
7. Slowly lower resistance and repeat.
8. Move quickly to leg press after final repetition.

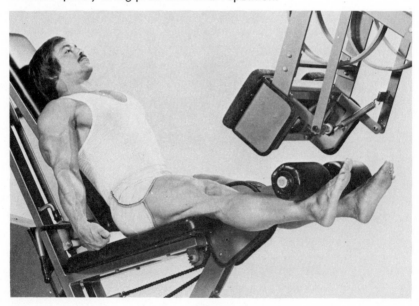

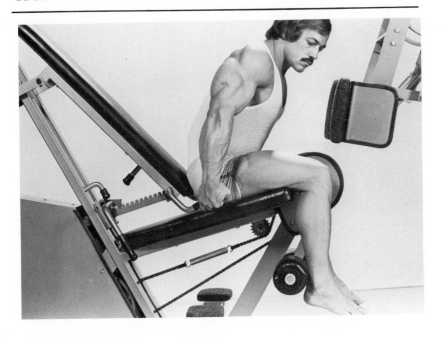

Leg Press

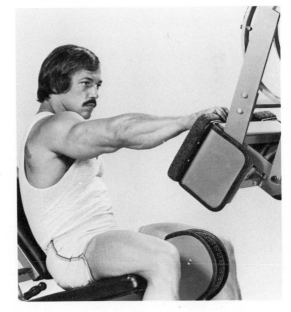

1. Flip down foot pads
   (above).

2. Sit erect and pull
   seat forward
   (right).

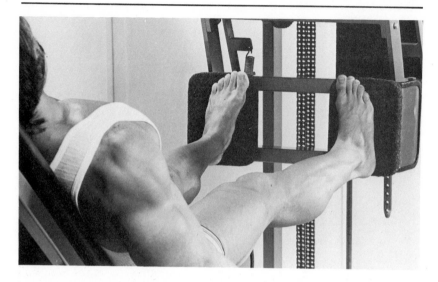

3. Place both feet on pads with toes pointed slightly inward.
4. Straighten both legs in a controlled manner.
5. Avoid tightly gripping handles and do not grit teeth or tense neck or face muscles.

6. Return to starting position and repeat.

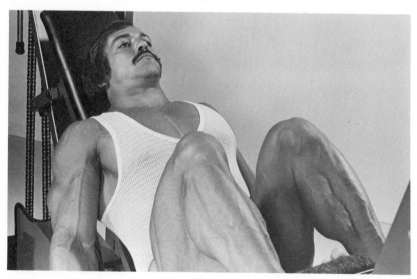

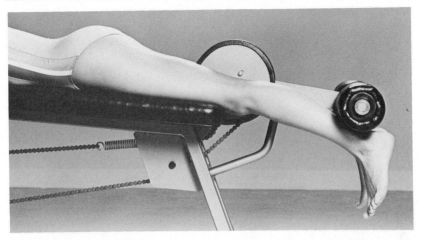

LEG CURL MACHINE

1. Lie face down on machine.
2. Place feet under roller pads with knees just over edge of bench.
3. Grasp handles to keep body from moving.

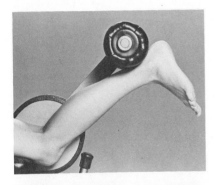

4. Curl legs and try to touch heels to buttocks.

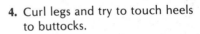

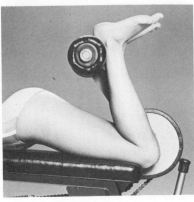

5. Lift buttocks to increase movement.
6. Pause at point of full muscular contraction.
7. Lower resistance slowly and repeat.

MULTI-EXERCISE MACHINE

Calf Raise

1. Adjust belt comfortably around hips.
2. Place balls of feet on first step and hands on front of carriage.
3. Lock knees and keep locked throughout movement.
4. Elevate heels as high as possible and try to stand on big toes.
5. Pause.

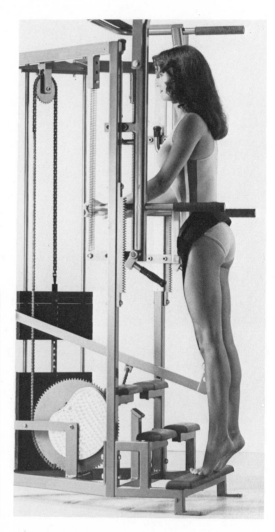

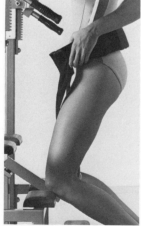

6. Lower heels slowly.
7. Stretch at bottom by lifting toes.
8. Repeat.

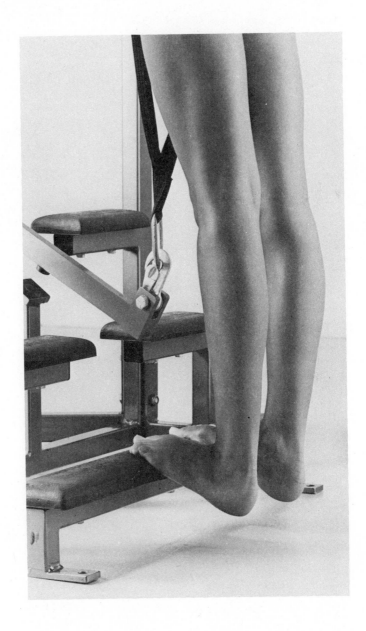

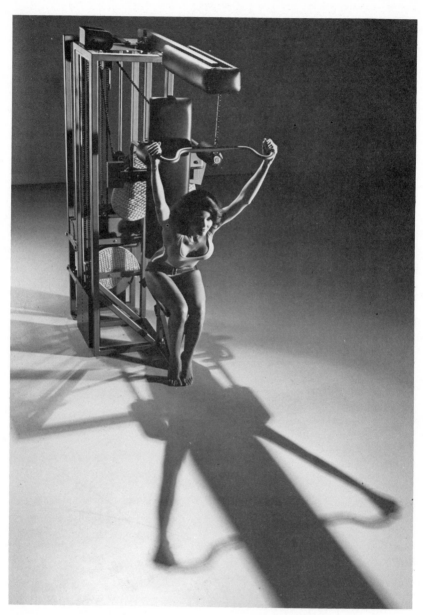

Behind neck/torso arm machine

CHAPTER SIX

back-torso

Strength-training experts have generally agreed that the full squat, more than any other barbell exercise, produces overall gains in size and strength. These results are not limited to the legs; overall gains are noticeable in the chest, back, and arms.

Since the squat is primarily a lower body exercise, it is no surprise that the greatest results are made in the legs. The upper body, however, does not respond to any type of barbell training as fast as the legs do to squats.

In the April 1970 *Iron Man* magazine, Arthur Jones published an article titled, "The Upper Body Squat." In this early Jones article, the athletic world was offered an exercise that would eventually revolutionize upper body training. "The upper body squat now exists," Jones wrote, "and it will do for the upper body just what squats have long done for the thighs."

Jones' upper body squat was the first successful method of providing direct exercise for the largest, strongest muscles of the upper body, the latissimus dorsi. These muscles join to the lower part of the spine and sweep up to the armpit where they are inserted into the upper arm bone. When the latissimus dorsi muscles contract they pull the upper arms from an overhead position down and around the shoulder axes. This rotational movement can take place with the upper arms in front of the body or on the sides of the body.

Several smaller back muscles also assist the latissimus dorsi in moving the upper arms. The most important of these muscles is the teres major.

Effectively placing the resistance on the elbows, as opposed to the hands as in conventional exercises, Jones' machine exposed the lats to direct resistance for the first time. "In six weeks," Jones wrote, "we built one subject's lats to a point that would have normally required at least two full years of training."

The original upper body squat was performed on a machine that would be considered crude today. Despite that consideration, Peary Rader, editor of the magazine, has said that Jones' "Upper Body Squat" article generated more mail than any other in the history of the publication. Jones included no photographs with his manuscript. It is open speculation whether that detracted from or actually stimulated interest in his new machine.

Today the Nautilus latissimus machines consist of the pullover/torso arm and behind neck/torso arm.

PULLOVER/TORSO ARM MACHINE

Pullover

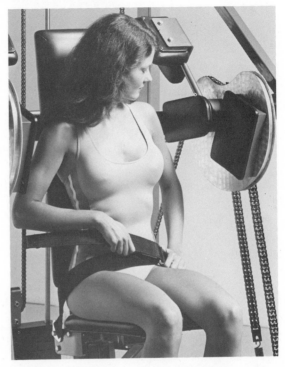

1. Adjust seat so shoulder joints are in line with axes of cams.
2. Assume erect position and fasten seat belt tightly.

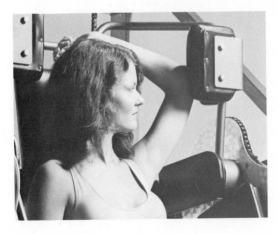

3. Leg press foot pedal until elbow pads are about eye level.
4. Place elbows on pads.

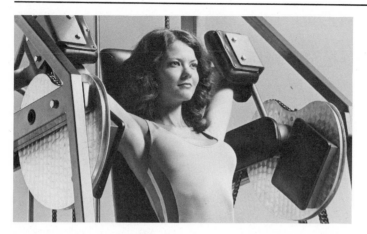

5. Remove legs from pedal and slowly rotate elbows as far back as possible.
6. Stretch.

7. Rotate elbows down until bar touches midsection.
8. Pause.
9. Return slowly to stretched position and repeat. After final repetition, immediately do pulldown.

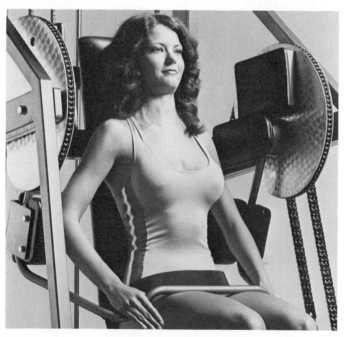

Torso Arm Pulldown

1. Lower seat to bottom for maximum stretch.

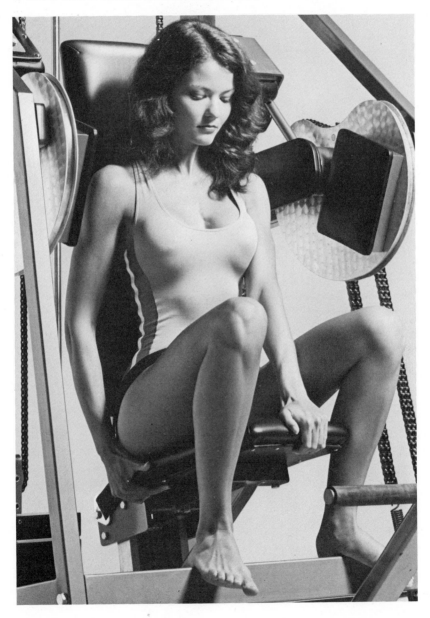

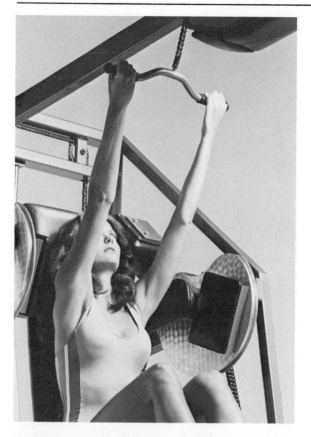

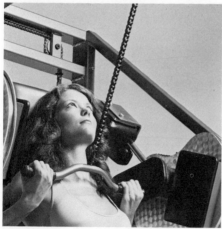

2. Grasp overhead bar with palms-up grip.
3. Keep head and shoulders against seat back.

4. Pull bar to chest.
5. Pause.
6. Return slowly to stretched position and repeat.

BEHIND NECK/TORSO ARM MACHINE

Behind Neck

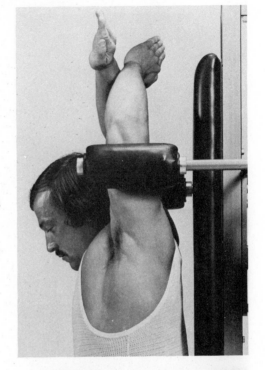

1. Adjust seat so shoulder joints are in line with axes of cams.
2. Fasten seat belt.
3. Place back of upper arms, triceps area, between padded movement arms.
4. Cross forearms behind neck.

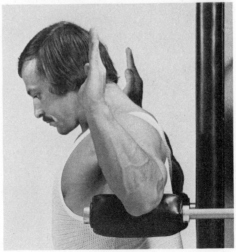

5. Move both arms downward until perpendicular to floor. Be careful not to bring arms or hands to front of body.
6. Pause.
7. Return slowly to crossed-arm position behind neck and repeat. After final repetition, immediately do behind neck pulldown.

Behind Neck Pulldown

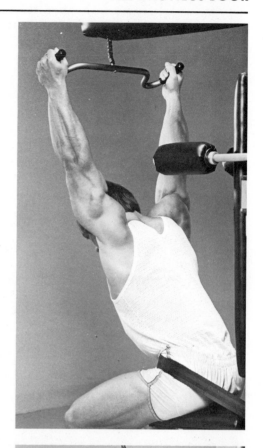

1. Lean forward and grasp
   overhead bar with
   parallel grip.

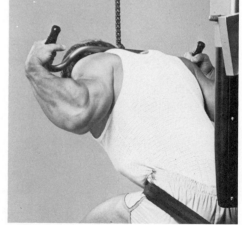

2. Pull bar behind neck,
   keeping elbows back.
3. Pause.
4. Return slowly to starting
   position and repeat.

MULTI-EXERCISE MACHINE
Side Bend

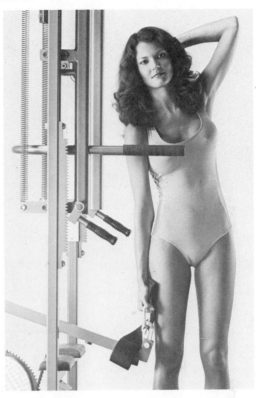

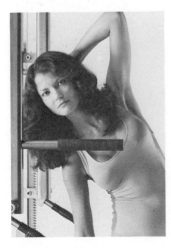

1. Attach belt or handle to movement arm.
2. Grasp handle in right hand with right shoulder facing machine.
3. Assume a standing position.
4. Place left hand on top of head.

5. Bend to the right side.
6. Return to standing position and repeat.
7. Change hands and do side bend to left side.

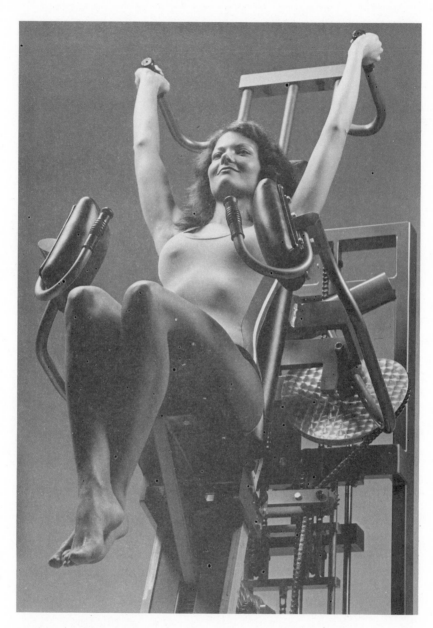

Double shoulder machine

CHAPTER SEVEN

shoulders

Shoulders are essential not only to a masculine appearance, but to success in athletics. Throwing a ball, swinging a bat, a tennis racquet, or a golf club are not feats for weak shoulders. The shoulder muscles are essential in swimming. In gymnastics and wrestling, the strength of the shoulders is often the determining factor in success. Even in sprinting, the limiting factor may not be leg speed, but arm speed, for the shoulder muscles play an important role in moving the arms.

Shoulders are also important to women. Being traditionally weak in the upper body, most women have more to gain from proper shoulder strengthening exercises than men. Bony shoulders not only look unattractive, especially in swim suits and low-cut gowns, but they can be the weak link in any activity that involves the arms.

The shoulders are the key to many whole-body movements. They allow for smooth coordination between the torso and arms. They are instrumental in transferring the whole bodily power to a specific object such as a racquet. The shoulder muscles are the element transferring body power into the arms, which along with hip rotation make a powerful swing. Stronger shoulders mean that an athlete can hit a ball hard and with expert efficiency.

Once you understand the essential role of the shoulders, you can see why it is important that they be kept strong at all times. Exceptional development of the shoulder muscles will give an individual an advantage over his opponents no matter what the activity. It will also add extra protection against various types of upper body injuries.

ANATOMY AND FUNCTION OF THE SHOULDERS

Movements of the shoulder joint are produced by eleven muscles. The most important of these muscles in size and shape is the deltoid. The deltoid, a triangular muscle, is on the shoulder with one angle pointing down the arm and the other two bent around the shoulder to front and rear.

The deltoid muscle is a single mass, but it is divided into three sections: anterior, middle, and posterior. Each is involved in moving the upper arm. The anterior deltoids lift the arms forward. The middle deltoids lift them sideways. The posterior deltoids lift them backwards.

Because of the separate functions of the deltoids, specific exercises should be used to develop all three sections. This assures symmetrical development and protects the shoulder joint from injury.

DOUBLE SHOULDER MACHINE

Lateral Raise

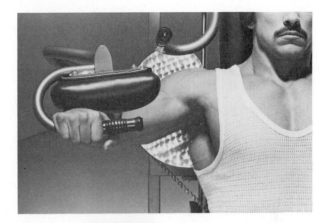

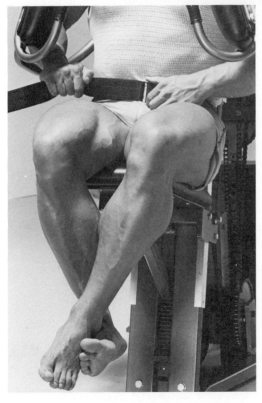

1. Adjust seat so shoulder joints with arms raised are in line with axes of cams.

2. Position thighs on seat, cross ankles, and fasten seat belt.

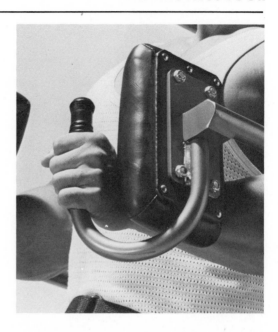

3. Pull handles back until
   knuckles touch pads.

4. Lead with elbows and raise both arms until parallel with floor.
5. Pause.
6. Lower resistance slowly and repeat. After final repetition, immediately
   do overhead press.

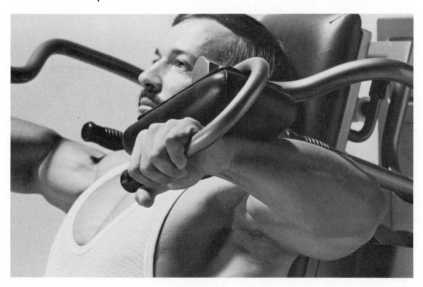

Overhead Press

1. Raise seat quickly for greater range of movement.

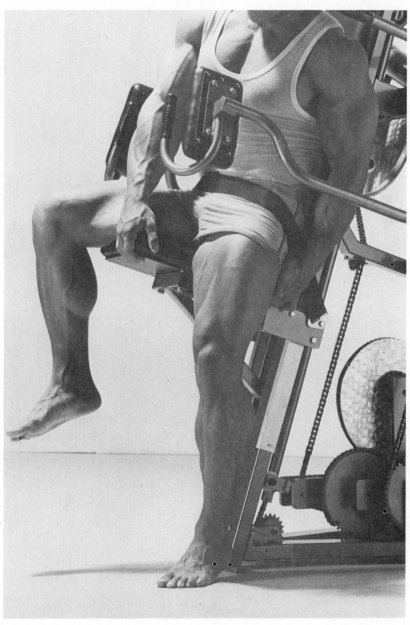

2. Grasp handles above shoulders.

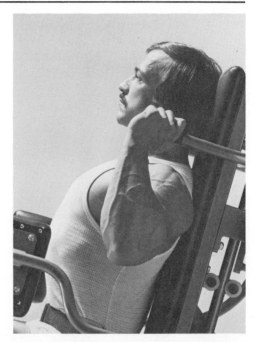

3. Press handles overhead while being careful not to arch the back.
4. Lower resistance slowly, keeping elbows wide, and repeat.

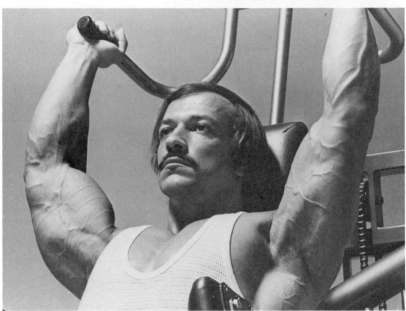

ROWING TORSO MACHINE

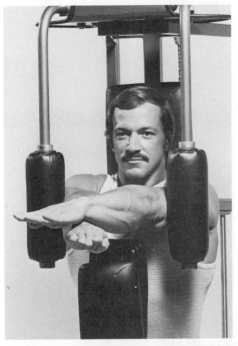

1. Sit with back toward weight stack.
2. Place arms between pads and cross arms.

3. Bend arms in rowing fashion as far back as possible.
4. Pause.
5. Return slowly to starting position and repeat.

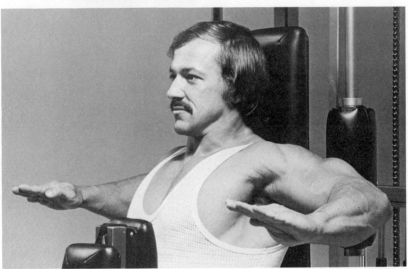

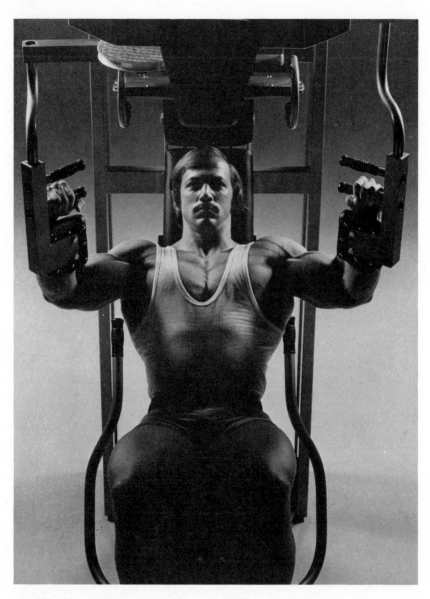

Double chest machine

CHAPTER EIGHT

chest

Men and women alike have long admired a firm, shapely chest. This may account for the fact that most Americans are dissatisfied with their chest development.

Every American woman is aware that she lives in a culture which places an extraordinary emphasis on female breasts. Men interested in exercise usually have at least two goals in mind: a big arm and a big chest. Regardless of sex, these individuals feel their chest is too small, too large, too flabby, too flat, or too weak—but seldom just right.

Until the Nautilus double chest machine was designed and built in 1973, no exercise worked the chest muscles without involving the weaker muscles of the upper arms. Conventional exercises for the chest, such as barbell bench presses and dumbbell flies, are dependent on the strength of the triceps. Since the triceps are much smaller and weaker than the pectoralis major muscles of the chest, the triceps fatigued long before the pectorals could be fully worked.

By placing the resistance on the elbows rather than the hands, the Nautilus double chest machine bypassed the weaker muscles of the arms. The pectoral muscles could be directly worked. Direct resistance for these muscles would now allow people to make significant progress in attaining a strong, shapely chest.

MUSCLES OF THE CHEST

Although there are numerous muscles surrounding the chest area, the pectoralis major is the most important. It is the large fan-shaped muscle lying across the front of the chest. One end of this muscle is attached to the sternum and the other to the front of the upper arm. When the pectoral muscles contract, they move the upper arms across the body. Up to this point, the male and female physical make-up is relatively the same. However, while a woman's breasts are attached to the pectoralis major muscles, they are not composed of muscle tissue. Breasts are composed of fatty tissue, milk glands, connective tissue, and blood vessels. The only muscles in the female breast are in the erectile portion of the nipple and they have no potential for development.

Little can be done to increase the size of the female breast, outside of hormone drugs, silicone injections, surgery, or a large increase or decrease in body fat. Proper exercise, however, can definitely expand and increase the strength and tone of the underlying and surrounding muscle structures. As a result, the breasts will become firmer so they protrude more or are carried higher on the chest. Loose skin will also become tauter from proper exercise, and posture will be improved. A woman's bustline will take on new shape and contours as a result of improved tone and strength in the chest muscles.

Men can improve the tone of the muscles of the chest and develop its muscular size and strength. This is mainly because certain hormones are present in greater quantities in the male than in the female.

DOUBLE CHEST MACHINE

Arm Cross

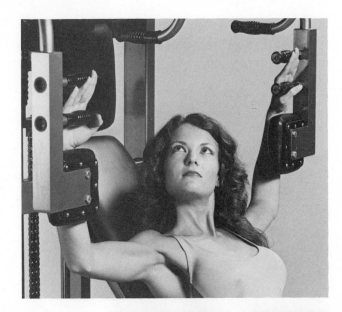

1. Adjust seat until shoulders, when elbows are together, are directly under axes of overhead cams.
2. Fasten seat belt.
3. Place forearms behind and firmly against movement arm pads.
4. Grasp handles, thumb should be around handle, and keep head against seat back.

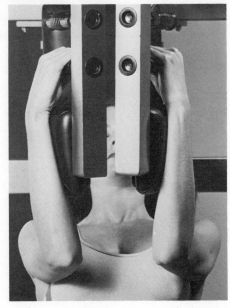

5. Push with forearms and try to touch elbows together in front of chest. (Movement can also be done one arm at a time in an alternate fashion.)
6. Pause.

7. Lower resistance slowly and repeat. After final repetition, immediately do decline press.

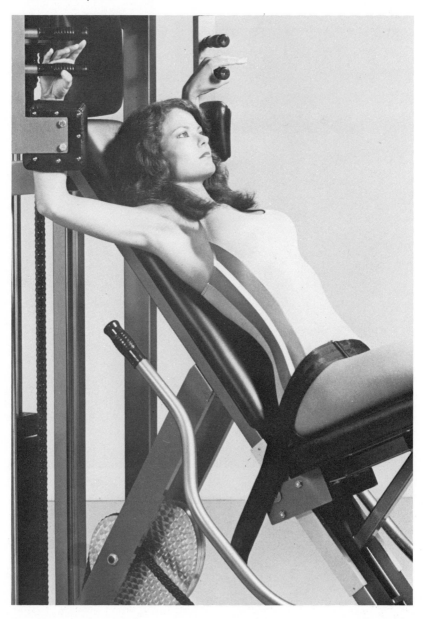

Decline Press

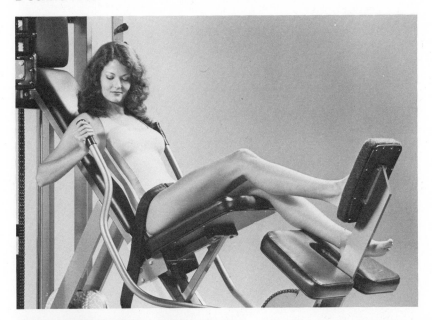

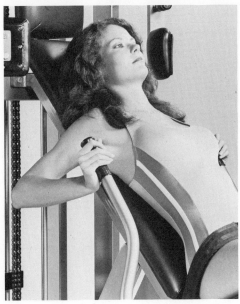

1. Use foot pedal to raise handles into starting position.
2. Grasp handles with parallel grip.

3. Keep head back and torso erect.
4. Press bars forward in controlled fashion.
5. Lower resistance slowly, keeping elbows wide.
6. Stretch in the bottom position and repeat pressing movement.

MULTI-EXERCISE MACHINE

Parallel Dip (negative only with or without weight belt)

1. Adjust carriage to proper level. It is important to allow ample stretch in bottom position.

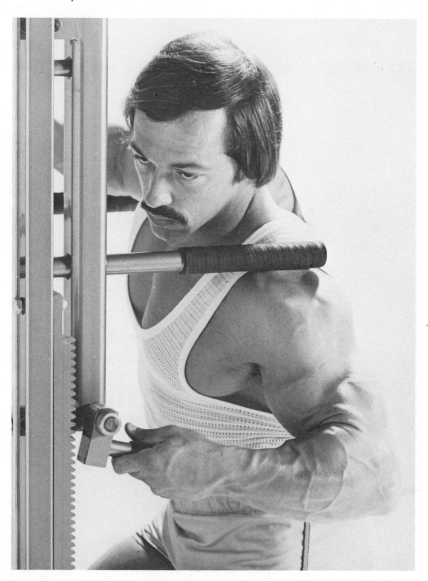

2. Climb steps.
3. Lock elbows and bend legs.

4. Lower body slowly by bending arms (8–10 seconds).
5. Stretch at bottom position.
6. Climb up and repeat.

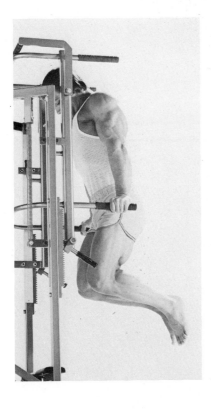

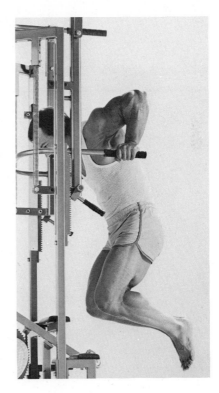

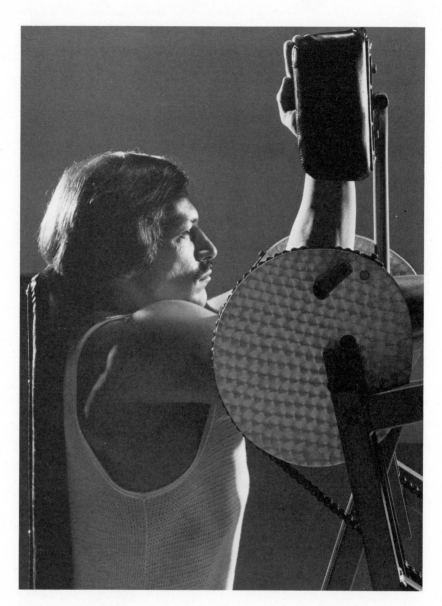

Multi-triceps machine

CHAPTER NINE

arms

In 1973, Arthur Jones still believed that the previous generation of bodybuilders, those of the 1940s and 1950s, were rational men. After a number of such men had appeared at the Nautilus headquarters, however, Jones was beginning to wonder. One Mr. America candidate of the 1940s whose massive arms were a special status symbol in his heyday arrived. Even the great Sergio Oliva, whose arms were as big as his own head, exclaimed, "They're too big!" when shown a picture of the man's arms.

A young athlete on the Nautilus staff, anxious to learn his scientific techniques, asked the man simply, "What is the secret to building big arms?"

Without hesitation the soft-spoken man with the enormous arms answered, "You know, young man, that the muscles are comprised mostly of water. Therefore you must train your arms with the heaviest weight possible, then you must drink at least a gallon of water during and just after your workout, and finally you must pray that God will direct the water to your arms."

Arthur Jones is now convinced that bodybuilders of the 1940s and 1950s incorporated as much myth and superstition in their training as current bodybuilders do.

OLD MYTHS STILL LINGER

One prominent myth is the belief that with the so-called bombing and blitzing methods made popular by bodybuilding magazines, one can develop championship arms. Less than one percent of the male population in this country has the genetic potential to develop the arm size of a Mr. America winner. Anyone can build larger and stronger arms, but unless he has long muscle bellies in his biceps and triceps, really large muscular upper arms are an impossibility.

Even though many coaches and athletes are aware of the benefits of strength training for the arms, some still cling to the old myth about resistance exercise slowing coordination and speed of limbs. They still think that "muscle-bound" is an actual condition. Strength training will not make an individual slow and clumsy or muscle-bound. This has been proven by scientific research.

Another myth is the misunderstanding that muscles are made of protein, and to build large muscles a person must consume massive amounts of protein foods. (That 1940s Mr. America competitor was at least correct when he stated that most of a muscle is water. Seventy percent of a muscle is water and only 22 percent protein.) Even before a muscle is to be nourished, there must be growth stimulation at the basic cellular level. After puberty, growth stimulation occurs in almost direct proportion to the intensity of the exercise. High-intensity exercise results in maximum degrees of growth stimulation. This growth will occur if the stimulated muscle is allowed at least 48 hours of rest. Nutrition is very secondary to the high-intensity exercise and rest requirements. All the body requires is a few nutrients, which it can easily obtain from fat stores, and water.

MUSCLES OF THE ARMS

The upper arm is basically composed of two large muscles and thirteen smaller ones. These muscles cross the elbow joint and control its flexing and extending. Eight muscles contribute to flexion, seven to extension. The most important muscle of the elbow flexion is the biceps. The most important muscle of elbow extension is the triceps.

The biceps is the prominent muscle on the front side of the upper arm. It is a two-headed muscle made up of a long and a short head. The tendons at the top end cross the shoulder joint and are attached to the scapula. At the other end the tendons cross the elbow and are connected to the forearm just below the joint. The biceps cross two joints, the shoulder and the elbow.

The functions of the biceps are three-fold. It supinates the hand, flexes the elbow, and lifts the upper arm forward. In order for the biceps to contract fully, the hand must be supinated, the elbow must be bent, and the upper arm must be raised to ear level.

The triceps is on the back side of the upper arm, and as its name implies, has three separate heads: lateral, medial, and long. Like the biceps, the triceps tendons cross both the shoulder and the elbow joint.

The major function of the triceps is to straighten the elbow. It also assists in bringing the upper arm down from an overhead position. For the triceps to be fully contracted, the upper arm must be behind the torso as the elbow straightens.

Nineteen separate muscles make up the forearm. These muscles act on both the fingers and the wrist. The bulk of the musculature is concentrated in two masses just below the elbow joint. The mass on the outside is formed by the bellies of the extensor muscles. The inside mass of the forearm comes from the bellies of the flexor muscles.

The forearms are a very complex structure. Disregarding the flexion of the forearm against the upper arm, which is primarily caused by the biceps of the upper arm, the functions of the forearm are as follows: supination of the hand, pronation of the hand, gripping, extending the fingers, and bending the hand in four separate directions.

BICEPS/TRICEPS MACHINE

Biceps Curl

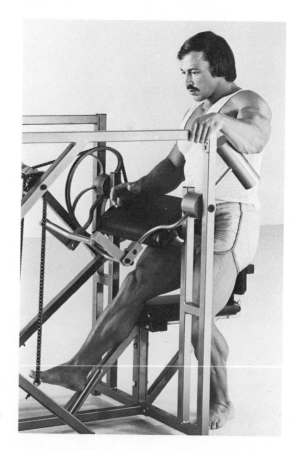

1. Enter machine from left side.

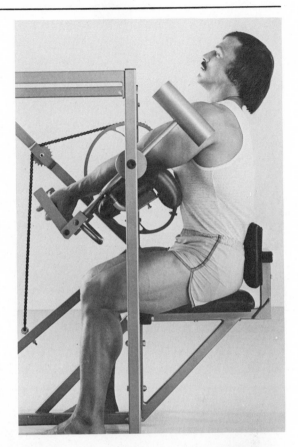

2. Place elbows on pad and in line with axis of cam.
3. Grasp bar with hands together and palms up. Lean back at full extension to ensure stretching.

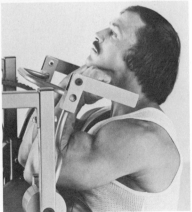

4. Curl bar smoothly until it reaches neck.
5. Pause.
6. Return slowly to stretched position and repeat.

Triceps Extension

1. Adjust seat position, with pads, if necessary, until shoulders are on same level as elbows.

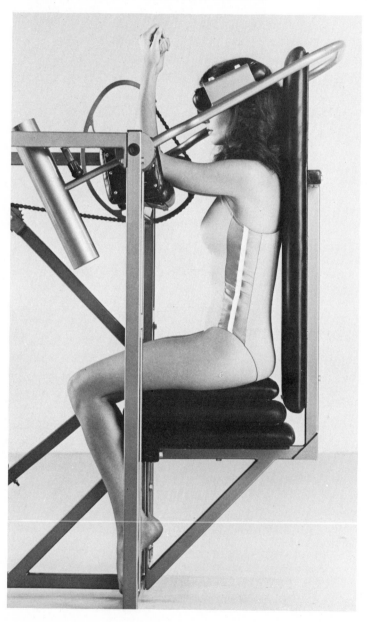

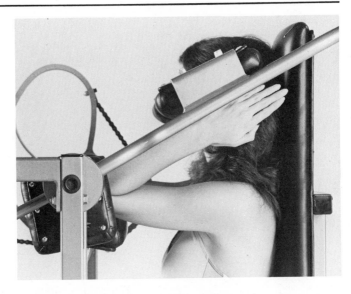

2. Place elbows in line with axis of cam, and
hands with thumbs up on pads.

3. Straighten arms smoothly.
4. Pause.
5. Return slowly to stretched position and repeat.

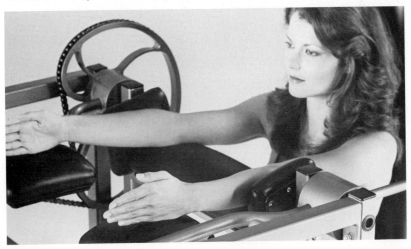

COMPOUND POSITION BICEPS MACHINE

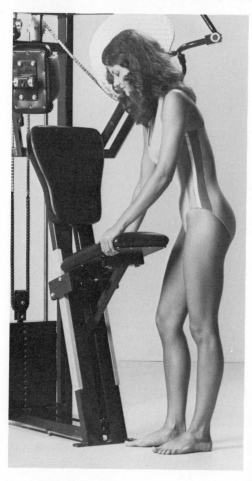

1. Adjust seat so elbows are in line with axes of cams.

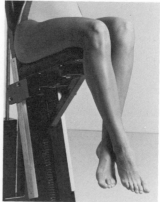

2. Place thighs on seat and cross ankles.

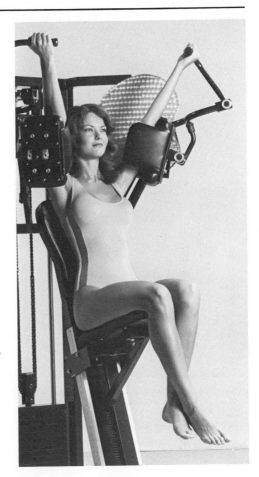

3. Extend arms and lightly
grasp handles.

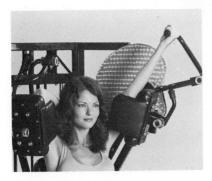

4. Curl one arm behind neck.
Movement arms can also be
curled together.
5. Pause.
6. Lower resistance slowly.
7. Repeat with other arm.

COMPOUND POSITION TRICEPS MACHINE

4. Extend arms smoothly, keeping elbows against pads.
5. Pause.
6. Return slowly to stretched position and repeat.

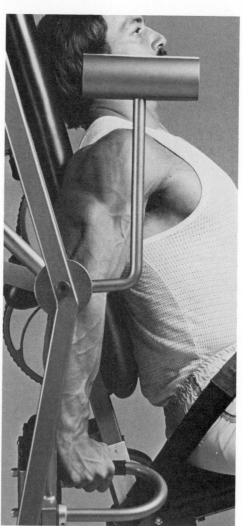

1. Adjust seat so elbows are in line with axis of cam.
2. Keep elbows against pads, head and shoulders against seat back, and thighs on seat.
3. Grasp handles lightly with sides of hands on pads.

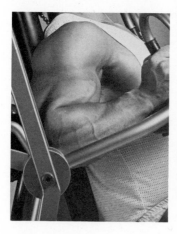

MULTI-BICEPS MACHINE—MOVEMENT-RESTRAINING STOP IN SIDE POSITION*

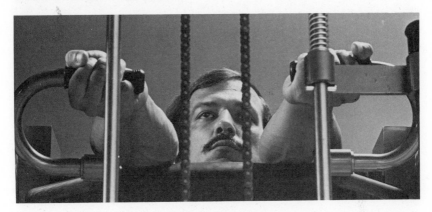

1. Place elbows on pads and in line with the axes of cams.
2. Place seat so shoulders are slightly lower than elbows. Machine can be used in at least eight different ways.

Two Arms Normal

1. Curl both arms to the contracted position.
2. Pause.
3. Lower slowly to the stretched position and repeat.

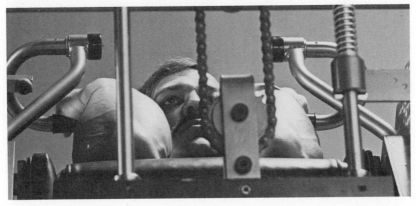

Movement-restraining stop in side and center positions is shown on page 106.

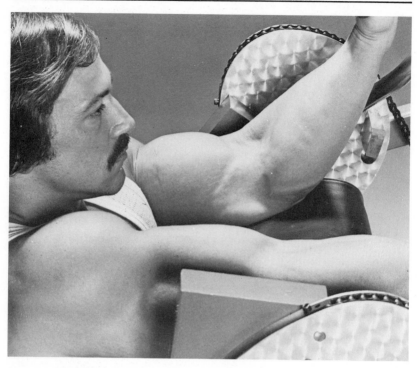

Two Arms Alternate

1. Do a complete repetition with one arm.
2. Do another complete repetition with the opposite arm.
3. Alternate back and forth until momentary muscular exhaustion.

Two Arms Duo/Poly

1. Bring both arms to the contracted position.
2. Holding one arm in the contracted position, lower the resistance with the opposite arm and curl the movement arm back to the contracted position.
3. Repeat with the other arm.

One Arm Normal

1. Work one arm to exhaustion, usually the nondominant arm first. An individual will be able to handle slightly more resistance with one arm than two.
2. Work the other arm to exhaustion.

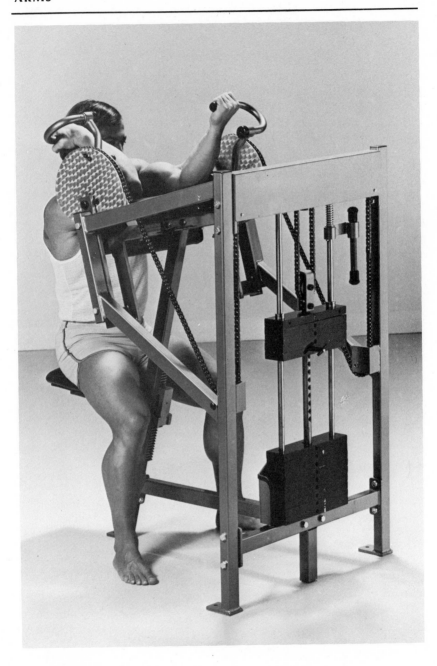

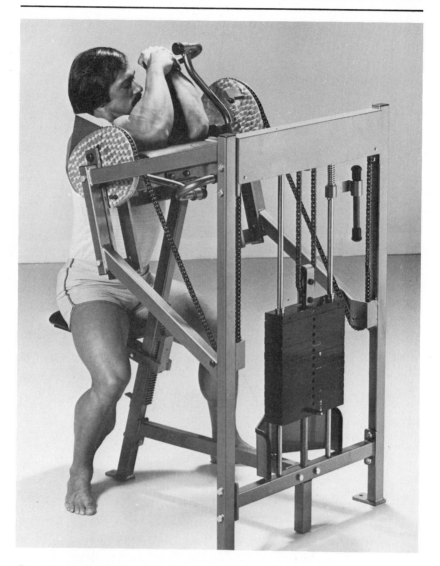

One Arm Negative Emphasized

1. Use the opposite arm for assistance in curling a heavier than normal weight.
2. Lower slowly the resistance with one arm.
3. Continue in this fashion until the biceps is unable to control the downward movement.
4. Repeat the procedure with the other arm.

MULTI-BICEPS MACHINE—MOVEMENT-RESTRAINING STOP IN CENTER POSITION

Infimetric

Remove the selector pin from the weight stack. Curl both arms to the mid-range position or until contact is made with the movement-restraining stop. In order for one arm to bend, the other arm must unbend or straighten. The trainee can vary the force by resisting more or less with the unbending arm. The movement should be smooth and steady with no dropping of the weight.

Position for infimetric, isometric, and akinetic exercise.

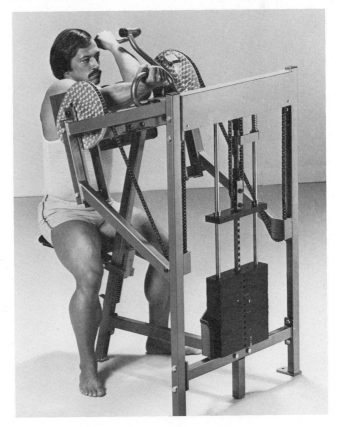

Isometric

Same procedure as infimetric, except do not permit movement of the unbending arm. Since an individual is 40-percent stronger negatively than positively, the negative or unbending arm is always able to prevent movement in the positive arm. It is possible, therefore, to provide an isometric or static condition at any point along the range of movement of the machine.

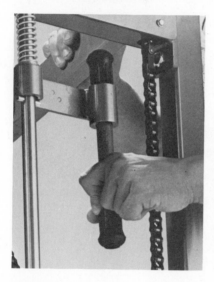   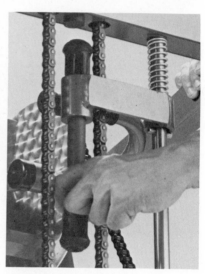

Movement-restraining stop in the side position.   Movement-restraining stop in the center position.

Akinetic

The primary difference between infimetric and akinetic is that in infimetric the selector pin is not used, while in akinetic a pre-determined amount of resistance is used. With infimetric training, it is very difficult to estimate the amount of force that is being exerted during the movement. With akinetic training, however, a medium resistance is selected and although a trainee can exert more force, any time he exerts less force, the weight stack drops noticeably.

MULTI-TRICEPS MACHINE—MOVEMENT-RESTRAINING STOP IN SIDE POSITION

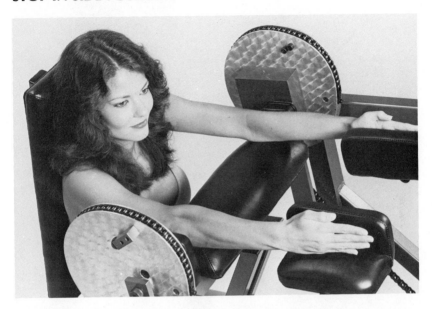

1. Adjust seat so shoulders are slightly lower than elbows.
2. Place sides of hands on movement arms and elbows on pad and in line with the axes of cams. Machine can be used in at least eight different ways.

Two Arms Normal *(above)*

1. Straighten both arms to the contracted position.
2. Pause.
3. Lower slowly to the stretched position and repeat.

Two Arms Alternate *(following page, top)*
1. Do a complete repetition with one arm.
2. Do another complete repetition with the opposite arm.
3. Alternate back and forth until momentary muscular exhaustion.

Two Arms Duo/Poly *(following page, top)*
1. Straighten both arms to the contracted position.
2. Holding one arm in the contracted position lower the resistance with the opposite arm and return to the contracted position.
3. Repeat with the other arm.

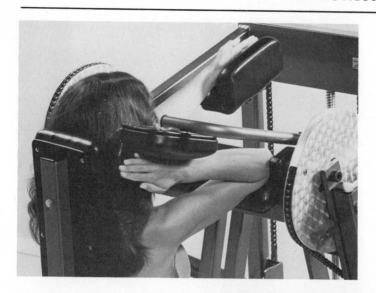

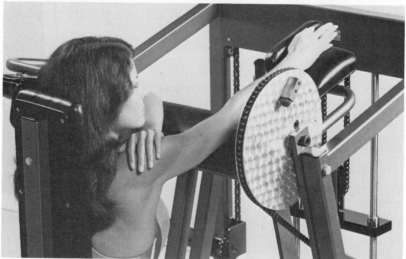

One Arm Normal

1. Work one arm to exhaustion, usually the non-dominant arm first. An individual will be able to handle slightly more resistance with one arm than with two.
2. Work the other arm to exhaustion.

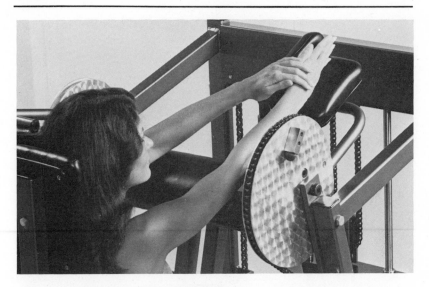

One Arm Negative Emphasized

1. Use the opposite arm for assistance in lifting a heavier than normal weight.
2. Lower slowly the resistance arm with one arm.
3. Continue in this fashion until the triceps is unable to control the downward movement.
4. Repeat the procedure with the other arm.

MULTI-TRICEPS MACHINE—MOVEMENT-RESTRAINING STOP IN CENTER POSITION

Infimetric

Remove the selector pin from the weight stack. Extend both arms to the mid-range position, or until contact is made with the movement-restraining stop. In order for one arm to straighten, the other arm must bend. The trainee can vary the force by resisting more or less with the bending arm. The movement should be smooth and steady with no dropping of the weight.

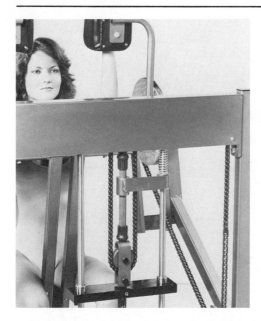

Movement-restraining stop in the center position.

Isometric

Same procedure as infimetric, except do not permit movement of the bending arm. Since an individual is 40-percent stronger negatively than positively, the negative arm is always able to prevent movement in the positive arm. It is possible, therefore, to provide an isometric or static contraction at any point along the range of movement of the machine.

Akinetic

The primary difference between infimetric and akinetic is that in infimetric the selector pin is not used, while in akinetic a pre-determined amount of resistance is used. With infimetric training, it is very difficult to estimate the amount of force that is being exerted during the movement. With akinetic training, however, a medium resistance is selected and although a trainee can exert more force, any time he exerts less force, the weight stack drops noticeably.

MULTI-EXERCISE MACHINE

Chin (negative only with or without weight belt)

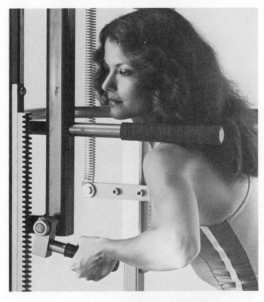

1. Place cross bar in forward position.
2. Adjust carriage to proper height. When standing on top step, chin should be barely over bar.

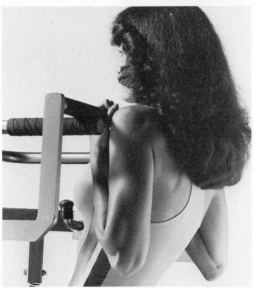

3. Grasp cross bar with palms up. Movement can also be done in a behind-neck fashion by using parallel grip.
4. Climb steps.
5. Place chin over bar, elbows by sides, and legs bent.

6. Lower body (8–10 seconds).

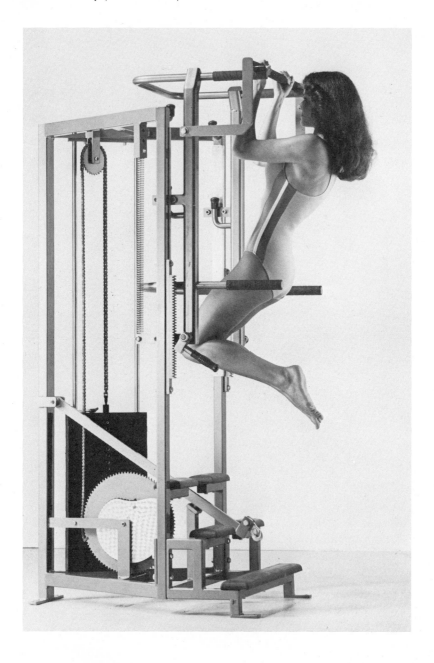

7. Stretch at bottom position.
8. Climb up and repeat.

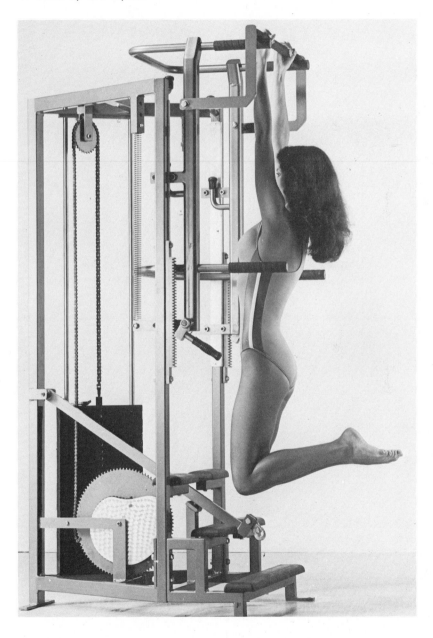

Wrist Curl

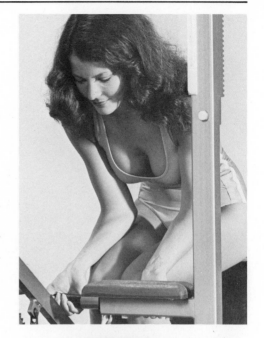

1. Sit in front of machine, using small bench or chair, with toes under first step.
2. Attach small bar directly to movement arm.
3. Grasp handles in a palms-up fashion. Palms-down grip should also be used.

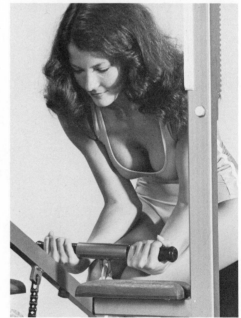

4. Place forearms firmly against thighs. Only hands should move.
5. Curl handles upward.
6. Pause.
7. Lower resistance slowly and repeat.

Triceps Extension

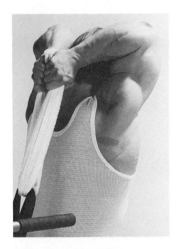

1. Loop a lightweight towel through weight belt.
2. Grasp one end of towel in each hand. Stand and face away from machine. Arms should now be bent with elbows by ears.
3. Adjust grip on towel until weight stack is separated.

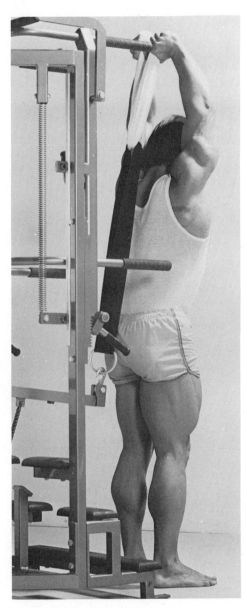

4. Straighten arms in a very smooth fashion.
5. Pause.
6. Lower resistance slowly and repeat.

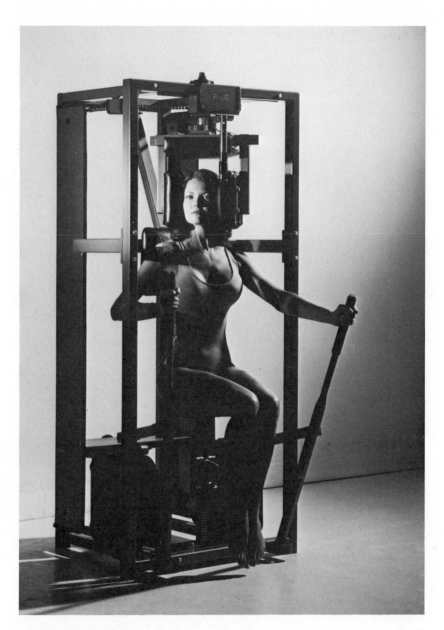

Rotary neck machine

CHAPTER TEN

neck

No part of the body is taken for granted as much as the neck, but few muscles are more important.

The neck acts as a natural barometer for the body. Illness shows its effect by giving the neck a haggard, drawn look. The healthy person has fullness of neck that adds confidence to his appearance.

Football players, wrestlers, boxers, and other athletes know the importance of a powerful neck. It acts as a shock absorber, preventing injury to the head, shoulders, and neck itself. The neck enables the athlete to use his head physically as well as mentally. Strong neck muscles permit such violent actions as blocking and tackling in football, and bridging in wrestling. Athletes have survived serious automobile accidents because of the strength and development of their necks.

Whiplash and other neck injuries happen to thousands of people every week as a result of minor accidents. Many of

117

these injuries would not have happened if the victim had had a strong neck. Even in simple calisthenic-type exercises or weekend sporting activities, there are many cases of preventable stiff necks and pulled neck muscles.

A strong neck is not only a safeguard against injury, but an addition to personal appearance. A thin, scrawny neck stands out conspicuously even in the best built man or woman.

In bodybuilding magazines some so-called experts advise against neck work. They reason that a large neck will detract from shoulder width. This makes about as much sense as never working the lower body so the upper body will look bigger. One of the real values of bodybuilding comes from all-over symmetry, from the pleasing development of all major muscle groups. Fortunately, for those who want to strengthen the neck, that part of the body responds quickly to proper exercise.

When they are provided with direct exercise, the muscles of the neck are perhaps the easiest in the body to develop. Until the advent of the Nautilus neck machines, there was no practical method of providing such direct exercise. Most of the available exercises were clumsy, difficult to perform, uncomfortable, and sometimes even dangerous. As a result, this important section of the body has been largely ignored.

ANATOMY OF THE NECK

When man assumed the upright position, the huge muscles of the nape of the neck atrophied. Now man balances his head, weighing about 14 pounds, upon seven small cervical vertebrae. The only restraining elements that oppose sudden movements of the neck are the strength and integrity of the cervical vertebrae, the spinal ligaments, and the neck muscles. It is essential, therefore, to strengthen and develop this protective musculature.

At least 15 small and medium sized muscles make up the

majority of the neck's mass. These muscles are capable of producing movement in seven different directions:

1.   Elevating the shoulders
2.   Bending the head toward the chest
3.   Drawing the head backward
4.   Bending the head down toward the right shoulder
5.   Bending the head down toward the left shoulder
6.   Twisting the head to look over the right shoulder
7.   Twisting the head to look over the left shoulder

When full-range exercise is provided for those seven functions, the response of the neck muscles is immediate. The neck responds quickly to exercise because its muscles are exposed to so little hard work. Development of the neck muscles therefore is not a matter of years, but of weeks.

4-WAY NECK MACHINE

Anterior Flexion

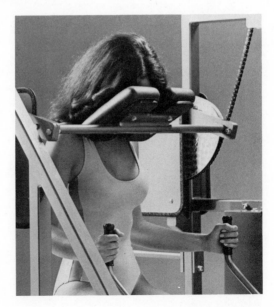

1. Face machine.
2. Adjust seat so nose is in center of pads.
3. Stabilize torso by lightly grasping handles.
4. Move head smoothly toward chest.
5. Pause.
6. Return slowly to stretched position and repeat.

Posterior Extension

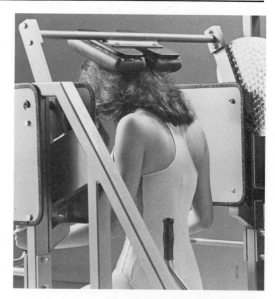

1. Turn body in machine until back of head contacts center of pads.
2. Stabilize torso by lightly grasping handles.
3. Extend head as far back as possible.
4. Pause.
5. Return slowly to stretched position and repeat.

Lateral Contraction

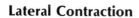
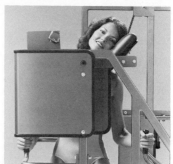

1. Turn body in machine until left ear is in center of pads.
2. Stabilize torso by lightly grasping handles.
3. Move head toward left shoulder.
4. Pause.
5. Keep shoulders square.
6. Return slowly to stretched position and repeat.
7. Reverse procedure for right side.

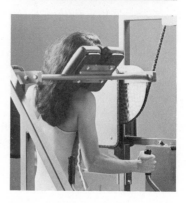

ROTARY NECK MACHINE

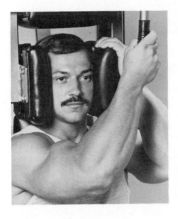

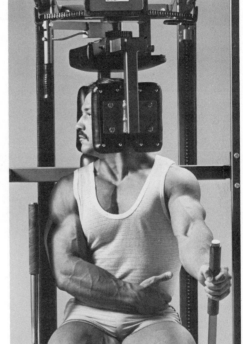

1. Sit facing away from machine.
2. Move head between pads.
3. Adjust head pads to a snug position by pulling overhead lever from right to left.

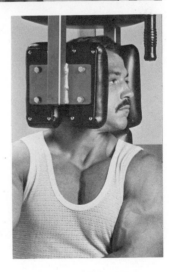

4. Push the hand levers to provide the resistance in this machine. Negative-only exercise can be provided by pressure on either hand lever, which will force the head to turn. This turning pressure is resisted by the neck muscles.
5. Push with the right hand lever, or pull with the left hand lever, to force the neck and head to rotate to the left or vice versa.

6. Perform six negative-only style repetitions to the right and six negative-only style repetitions to the left in an alternate fashion.
7. Release head pads by pulling overhead lever from left to right.

NECK AND SHOULDER MACHINE

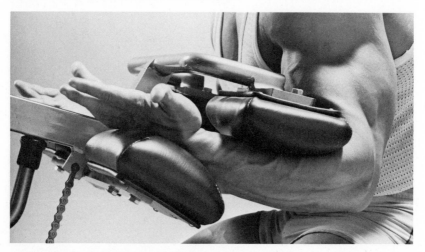

1. Place forearms between pads while seated.
2. Keep palms open and back of hands pressed against bottom pads.

3. Straighten torso until weight stack is lifted. The seat may be raised with elevation pads *(below, left)*.
4. Shrug shoulders smoothly as high as possible. Keep elbows by sides. Do not lean back *(below, right)*.

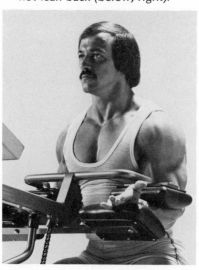

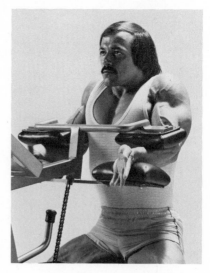

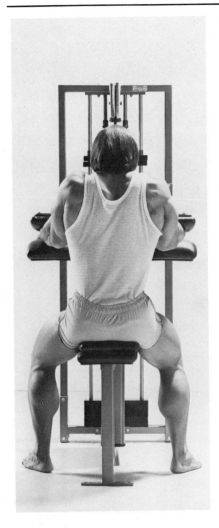

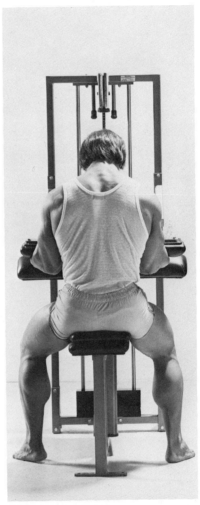

5. Pause.

6. Return slowly to stretched position and repeat.

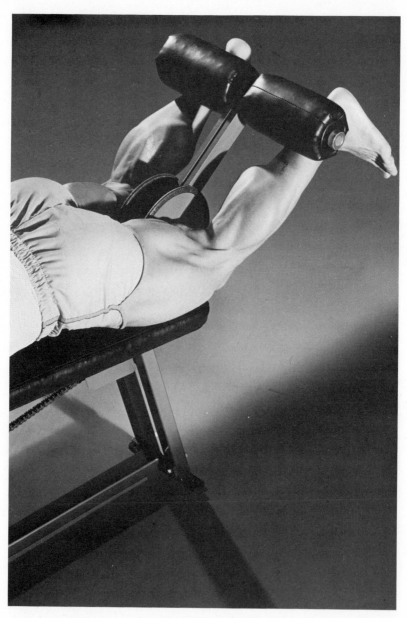

Leg curl machine

CHAPTER ELEVEN

nautilus routines

The following master listing of exercises, grouped by body part and equipment, is a summation of the last 7 chapters.

MASTER LISTING OF EXERCISES

Body Part	Nautilus Machine or Exercise
Buttocks	Hip and Back
	Leg Press
	Stiff-Legged Deadlift
Lower Back	Hip and Back
	Stiff-Legged Deadlift
Front Thigh	Leg Extension
	Leg Press
Back Thigh	Leg Curl
	Hip and Back
	Stiff-Legged Deadlift
	Leg Press

MASTER LISTING OF EXERCISES *(continued)*

Calves	Calf Raise
Back	Pullover/Torso Arm
	Pullover
	Torso-Arm Pulldown
	Behind Neck/Torso Arm
	Behind Neck
	Behind Neck Pulldown
	Neck and Shoulder
Shoulders	Double Shoulder
	Lateral Raise
	Overhead Press
	Rowing Torso
Chest	Double Chest
	Arm Cross
	Decline Press
	Pullover
Upper Arms	Compound Position Biceps Curl
	Biceps Curl (plateloading)
	Multi-Biceps Curl
	Compound Position Triceps Curl
	Triceps Extension (plateloading)
	Multi-Triceps Extension
Forearms	Wrist Curl
	Reverse Wrist Curl
Waist	Pullover
	Side Bend
Neck	4-Way Neck
	Rotary Neck
	Neck and Shoulder

TRIED AND PROVED ROUTINES

The following routines have been successfully used with men and women, athletes and non-athletes. If certain Nautilus machines are not available, substitutions can be made.

Abbreviations Used in Describing the Exercises and Styles of Training

(POTA)—Pullover/Torso-Arm Machine

(BNTA)—Behind Neck/Torso-Arm Machine

(DS)—Double Shoulder Machine

(DC)—Double Chest Machine

(ME)—Multi-Exercise Machine

(NO)—Negative-only exercise: the positive portion of an exercise movement is performed by assistants, or by the trainee's legs, as a heavier than normal weight is slowly lowered by the trainee.

(NA)—Negative-accentuated exercise: the trainee lifts the resistance with two limbs and slowly lowers with one limb.

(NE)—Negative-emphasized exercise: a lighter-than-normal weight is used on the positive part of the movement. Additional resistance is then provided on the negative phase by an assistant pressing down on the weight stack.

I	II
Basic Nautilus Workout	*Basic Nautilus Workout*
1. Hip and Back	1. Hip and Back
2. Leg Extension	2. Leg Extension
3. Leg Press	3. Leg Curl
4. Leg Curl	4. Calf Raise (ME)
5. Pullover (POTA)	5. Behind Neck (BNTA)
6. Pulldown (POTA)	6. Behind Neck Pulldown (BNTA)
7. Lateral Raise (DS)	7. Dip (ME)
8. Overhead Press (DS)	8. Rowing Torso
9. Neck and Shoulder	9. Triceps Extension
10. Arm Cross (DC)	10. Biceps Curl
11. Decline Press (DC)	11. Rotary Neck
12. 4-Way Neck	12. Neck and Shoulder

III

Basic
Nautilus Workout

1. Leg Curl
2. Leg Extension
3. Hip and Back
4. Calf Raise (ME)
5. Pullover (POTA)
6. Overhead Press (DS)
7. Chin (ME)
8. Dip (ME)
9. Side Bend (ME)
10. Rowing Torso
11. Wrist Curl (ME)
12. Reverse Wrist Curl (ME)

IV

Basic
Nautilus Workout

1. Hip and Back
2. Leg Extension
3. Leg Press
4. Leg Curl
5. Calf Raise (ME)
6. Lateral Raise (DS)
7. Overhead Press (DS)
8. Pullover (POTA)
9. Pulldown (POTA)
10. Arm Cross (DC)
11. Decline Press (DC)
12. Neck and Shoulder

V

Basic
Nautilus Workout

1. Leg Extension
2. Leg Press
3. Leg Curl
4. Hip and Back
5. Behind Neck (BNTA)
6. Chin (ME)
7. Decline Press (DC)
8. Rowing Torso
9. Multi-Triceps Extension
10. Compound Position Biceps
11. 4-Way Neck
12. Rotary Neck

VI

Basic
Nautilus Workout

1. Leg Press
2. Leg Extension
3. Stiff-Legged Deadlift (ME)
4. Calf Raise (ME)
5. Leg Curl
6. Lateral Raise (DS)
7. Pullover (POTA)
8. Decline Press (DC)
9. Wrist Curl (ME)
10. Reverse Wrist Curl (ME)
11. Neck and Shoulder
12. 4-Way Neck

VII

*Negative
Nautilus Workout*

1. Leg Extension (NA)
2. Leg Press (NA)
3. Leg Curl (NA)
4. Hip and Back (NA)
5. Pullover (NO)
6. Chin (NO)
7. Lateral Raise (NO)
8. Overhead Press (NO)
9. Neck and Shoulder
10. Dip (NO)

VIII

*Negative
Nautilus Workout*

1. Hip and Back (NA)
2. Leg Curl (NE)
3. Leg Press (NE)
4. Leg Extension (NE)
5. Rowing Torso (NE)
6. Decline Press (NO)
7. Pullover (NA)
8. Overhead Press (NA)
9. 4-Way Neck (NO)
10. Rotary Neck (NO)

IX

*Nautilus
Pre-Exhaustion Workout*

1. Leg Curl
2. Hip and Back
3. Stiff-Legged Deadlift
   (ME)
---
4. Leg Extension
5. Leg Press
---
6. Pullover (POTA)
7. Behind Neck (BNTA)
8. Behind Neck Pulldown
   (BNTA)
---
9. Triceps Extension (ME)
10. Dip (NO)
---
11. Biceps Curl
12. Chin (ME)

X

*Nautilus
Pre-Exhaustion Workout*

1. Leg Curl
2. Leg Extension
3. Leg Press
---
4. Behind Neck Pulldown
   (BNTA)
5. Behind Neck (BNTA)
6. Chin (NO)
---
7. Decline Press (DC)
8. Arm Cross (DC)
9. Dip (NO)
---
10. Side Bend (ME)
11. Trunk Curl
12. Pullover (POTA)

In routines **IX** and **X** rest only between exercises separated by a rule.

XI

Nautilus
Push and Pull Workout

1. Leg Press
2. Leg Curl
3. Leg Extension
4. Hip and Back
5. Overhead Press (DS)
6. Chin (ME)
7. Decline Press (DC)
8. Behind Neck Pulldown
   (BNTA)
9. Dip (ME)
10. Pullover (POTA)
11. Triceps Extension
12. Biceps Curl

XII

Nautilus
Push and Pull Workout

1. Hip and Back
2. Leg Extension
3. Leg Curl
4. Leg Press
5. Chin (ME)
6. Dip (ME)
7. Behind Neck (BNTA)
8. Overhead Press (DS)
9. Neck and Shoulder
10. Rotary Neck
11. Side Bend (ME)
12. 4-Way Neck

XIII

Nautilus
Change-of-Pace Workout

1. Overhead Press (DS)
2. Chin (ME)
3. Decline Press (DC)
4. Pullover (POTA)
5. Dip (ME)
6. Rowing Torso
7. Leg Extension
8. Leg Curl
9. Compound Position
   Triceps
10. Compound Position
    Biceps
11. Stiff-Legged Deadlift
    (ME)

XIV

Nautilus
Change-of-Pace Workout

1. Leg Press (Seat back)
2. Pullover (POTA)
3. Leg Press (Seat close)
4. Behind Neck (BNTA)
5. Calf Raise (ME)
6. Side Bend (ME)
7. Dip (ME)
8. Triceps Extension
9. Chin (ME)
10. Biceps Curl

IMPORTANT NOTE:

Three new Nautilus machines are being produced in 1980, Hip Abduction-Adduction, Abdominal/Hip Flexion, and Rotary Torso. Any or all of these machines can be alternated with other Nautilus equipment. The selection of exercises should not exceed 12 in any one workout, however.

CHOOSING A WORKOUT

If you're just beginning Nautilus training, you should start with Basic Nautilus Workout I. This workout should be performed three times a week for at least a month. After the first month, start alternating I with II, III, IV, V, and VI. After three more months of training, you should perform one negative workout per week. The other two workouts should come from the basic group. After several months of negative workouts, any of the other workouts can be used.

SPECIAL CONSIDERATIONS

Athletes

Under ideal circumstances, the athlete analyzes the specific sport or activity to determine the major muscle groups involved. The next step is to work those muscles throughout a full range of possible movement.

Almost all sports involve the contraction of every major muscle group in the body. All athletes, therefore, should use the same Nautilus routines. The program that produces excellent results for a football player will produce the same results for a basketball, baseball, soccer, and tennis player, or any other athlete.

It is a mistake to assume that the stronger the athlete becomes, the more exercise he needs. You should never perform over 12 exercises, and only one set of each, in any one workout. For many advanced, stronger athletes, the total number of exercises must be reduced to 10, or even to 8. Nautilus sessions should not be performed more than three times a week. Even this number may have to be reduced. The stronger the athlete becomes, the *less* exercise he needs.

In-season Nautilus training for an athlete merits special consideration. Too many athletes make the mistake of developing high levels of strength during the off-season and gradually losing that level during the season. To increase or even maintain muscular strength during the season, athletes must train hard at least once every four days. Steady progress can be made on a twice-a-week program.

Most in-season Nautilus training should be limited to twice a week. Usually the athletes who play a significant role during the game are trained the next day and again three days later. Training the day following the game eliminates much of the after-game soreness. The athletes who get little or no playing time during the game should continue training hard three times a week.

Women

Women have the same kind and number of muscles as men. The only difference between the training of a man and a woman is the amount of resistance on the Nautilus machine. Generally speaking, women will handle less weight than men. The training principles and program organization should be exactly the same for women as for men.

10 to 14 Age Group

Muscular strength is an important factor for the 10 to 14 age group for several reasons. First, strength provides the power behind all bodily movement. Second, it plays an important role in protecting the young from injury. Stronger muscles, of course, increase strength and joint stability.

A properly conducted Nautilus training program produces the following results for the 10 to 14 age group:

1. Increased muscular strength
2. Stronger ligaments, tendons, and connective tissues
3. Improved flexibility
4. Stronger bones
5. Increased heart-lung efficiency
6. Better protection against injury
7. Improved coordination
8. Faster speed of movement

Nautilus training of both boys and girls before puberty, and girls after puberty, produces little muscular development. The dominant masculinizing hormone, testosterone, is not secreted in large enough amounts in women to affect growth. Large muscular size from exercise, therefore, is only possible in males after puberty.

Prior to the age of about 10, most children will profit more by learning and practicing basic movement skills such as throwing, kicking, tumbling, climbing, jumping, and swinging. After the age of 10, however, properly conducted Nautilus training will benefit all children.

Basically, the same Nautilus training principles that have been used successfully with mature athletes apply to the 10 to 14 age group. It is very important that the young pay special attention to good form in all exercises. For them, supervision is very necessary.

Children under 5 feet in height and weighing less than 100 pounds should build a basic level of strength with freehand exercises before progressing to Nautilus machines. The following freehand routine is recommended as a starter program.

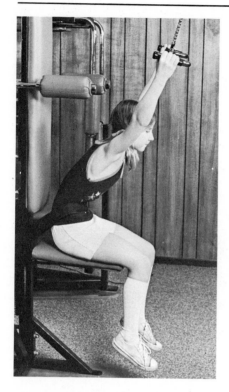

Many Nautilus machines can be used by children. Special attention should be given to slow, smooth movements. Here, a behind neck pulldown is performed by a 10-year-old girl.

1. Squat   4. Chin   7. Seated Dip
2. Reverse Leg Raise 5. Pushup   8. Trunk Curl
3. Calf Raise   6. Side Bend   9. Hand Resistance
                                        Against Neck

The young should start out by performing 8 repetitions of each exercise in good form. If that seems impossible on some movements, especially the chin, dip, or even the pushup, the following variations may be made.

In the chin, an adolescent can use his legs to help get his chin over the bar. Place a wooden box in front of the chinning bar. Have him step on the box and put his chin over the bar. Have him remove his feet and lower himself very slowly, in 6-8 seconds, then climb back and repeat. This is excellent exercise for the arms and back muscles. For building muscular strength, the lowering portion of the exercise is far more important than the raising part.

Dips on the parallel bars can be done in a similar manner. Have the boys and girls climb up, lock their arms, and lower themselves very slowly. This exercise works the chest, shoulders, and triceps.

In pushups, adolescents can use their knees and lower back to help straighten their arms. They should then slowly bend their arms until they touch the floor.

The squat can be done in one of two ways. Have the students bend their legs very slowly and smoothly, then stand up and repeat. They can work up to 10–15 seconds' lowering time on this exercise. Or, have them lower themselves on one leg, stand up on two legs, and lower themselves on the opposite leg. Some may need a chair to hold to for balance. For best results from these movements, only one set of 8–12 repetitions three times a week should be done.

Over 65 Age Group

The Census Bureau has estimated that there are 25 million people living in the United States over the age of 65. If present birth trends continue, an estimated 17 percent of the population will be 65 and older by the year 2030. The percentage now is 10.5. By 2030, over 50 million Americans will be 65 years or older.

Physical fitness can certainly improve life for those over 65. For those with normal health there is no better exercise than Nautilus training.

There are a few people in this age group, however, who should be precluded from vigorous exercise. Exercise may aggravate the condition of those who have acute arthritis, anemia, tuberculosis, severe kidney or liver diseases, or severe heart problems. In these cases a physician's recommendations should be rigidly adhered to.

A complete medical examination should, of course, be a prerequisite for anyone over 65 who is interested in exercise.

A month of supervised freehand exercises such as those described for adolescents would be appropriate to get sedentary muscles accustomed to progressive exercise. A Nautilus program could then be initiated with particular emphasis placed on slow, smooth, full-range movements. Results are often dramatic and very rewarding.

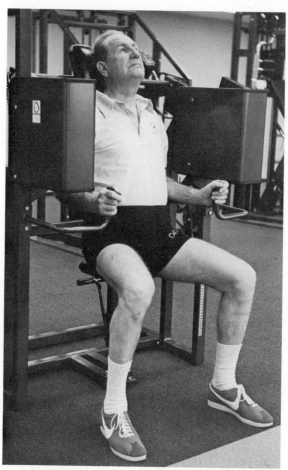

George Peterson (*above*), a 70-year-old businessman, and his wife, Pat (*opposite*), regularly train on Nautilus equipment at the Athletic Center of Atlanta, Georgia.

NAUTILUS FOR EVERYBODY

There is no age group that should be excluded from Nautilus exercise. It can enrich everybody's life. But it must be proper exercise—exercise properly organized, properly supervised, and properly performed.

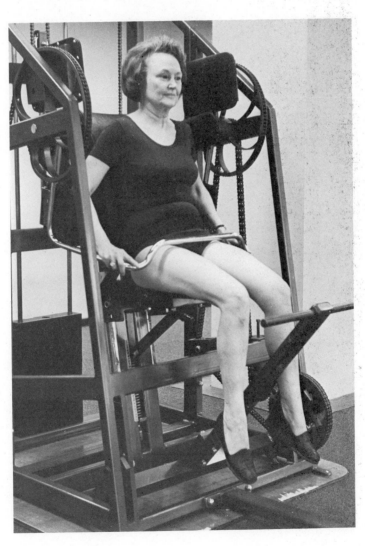

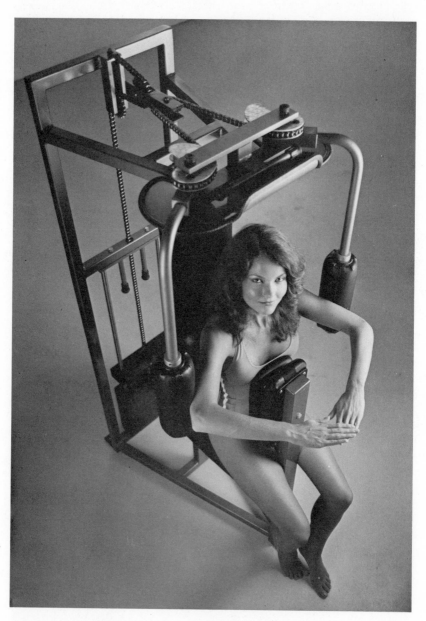

Rowing torso machine

CHAPTER TWELVE

questions and answers

The best way to fill in gaps and clear up areas of confusion seems to be the simple method of questions and answers. The following are answers to questions frequently asked in lecture sessions and by visitors to Nautilus Sports/Medical Industries.

ABDOMINAL MACHINE

Q. *Why is there no Nautilus abdominal machine?*

A. In July of 1980, Nautilus is introducing a combination Abdominal/Hip Flexion machine. The exercise with this machine is performed in a seated position with a padded belt across the thighs. As the hips are flexed, the trunk must be curled to meet the knees. A strong contraction is felt in the hip flexors and abdominals.

Until the Abdominal/Hip Flexion machine is available in

Nautilus fitness centers, the following free-hand exercise may be substituted:

Trunk curl: Lie face up on the floor with the hands behind the head. Bring heels up close to the buttocks and spread the knees. Try to curl the trunk to a sitting position. Only one-third of a standard situp can be performed in this manner. Slowly lower the trunk to the floor and repeat.

SITUPS AND LEG RAISES

Q. *Aren't situps and leg raises good abdominal exercises to supplement the Nautilus machines?*

A. The belief that situps and leg raises are abdominal exercises is a misconception. These movements work the hip flexors. The hip flexors connect the upper femur bones of the thighs to the lower lumbar region of the spine. When these muscles contract they pull the upper body to a sitting position, or pull the thighs toward the chest as in a leg raise. The abdominals are only mildly involved in a traditional situp or leg raise.

The previously described trunk curl isolates the hip flexors so the trainee does not inadvertently pull with them. It is important that the trainee not allow his feet and legs to be held down by a partner, strap, or other apparatus.

Another common misconception is that the midsection will be reduced if subjected to more repetitions than other body parts. Many people perform situps and leg raises by the hundreds in the mistaken belief that they will assist in burning fat and defining the waistline. Exercise for the midsection has no effect on fat loss in the waist. It cannot be emphasized too often that spot reduction is not possible. The abdominals should be treated as any other muscle group.

NEW NAUTILUS MACHINES

Q. *Does Nautilus plan on marketing other new machines?*

A. Yes! The Nautilus hip abduction-adduction machine went into production in April of 1980. Two important exercises are performed on this machine, abduction for the outer hips and adduction for the inner thighs. The Nautilus rotary torso machine is in the prototype stage. It provides stretching and contraction of many muscles of the midsection, such as the external obliques, internal obliques, erector spinae group, and deep posterior spinal group.

Hip Adduction (inner thighs)

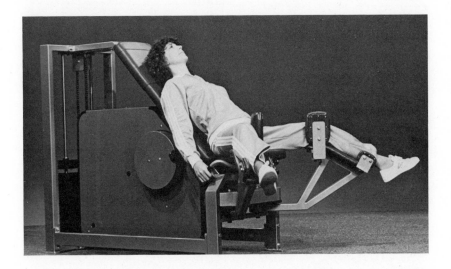

1. Adjust lever on right side of machine for range of movement. The farther the handle is pulled up, the greater the range of the machine.
2. Move thigh pads to inner position.
3. Sit in machine and place knees and ankles on movement arms in a spread-legged position. The inner thighs and knees should be firmly against the resistance pads.
4. Keep head and shoulders against seat back.
5. Grasp handles lightly.
6. Pull knees and thighs smoothly together.
7. Pause in knees-together position.
8. Return to stretched position and repeat.

Hip Abduction (outer hips)

1. Adjust lever on right side of machine until both movement arms are together.
2. Move thigh pads to outer position.
3. Sit in machine and place knees and ankles on movement arms. The outer thighs and knees should be firmly against resistance pads.
4. Keep head and shoulders against seat back.
5. Grasp handles lightly.
6. Spread knees and thighs to widest possible position.
7. Pause.
8. Return to knees-together position and repeat.

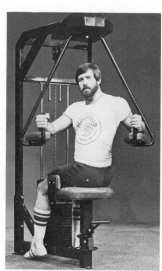

Prototype of rotary torso machine.

MUSCULAR GROWTH

Q. *What makes a muscle grow?*

A. Muscle growth is dependent on three things:

1. There must be growth stimulation within the body itself at the basic cellular level. After puberty, this is best accomplished by high-intensity Nautilus exercise.

2. The proper nutrients must be available for the stimulated cells. But providing large amounts of nutrients, in excess of what the body requires, does not promote growth of muscle fibers. The growth machinery within the cell must

be turned on. Muscle stimulation must always precede nutrition. If an athlete has stimulated muscular growth by high-intensity exercise, his muscles will grow given almost any reasonable diet and sufficient time.

3. Sufficient time, the third factor, means time spent in resting and recovering.

SIZE AND STRENGTH

Q. *What is the difference between muscular size and muscular strength?*

A. The strength of a muscle can be compared to that of a rope as both produce a pulling force in proportion to cross-sectional area. Since the length of a muscle is not changed by an increase in its volume, the cross-sectional area is in direct proportion to the volume. The volume of a muscle and its size are the same. Thus, the size of a muscle indicates its strength. Muscular growth always precedes an increase in strength.

PRE-STRETCHING

Q. *Where does pre-stretching fit into strength training?*

A. Pre-stretching is involved when a muscle is pulled into a position of increased tension prior to the start of a contraction. When a muscle is pre-stretched, a neurological signal is sent to the brain that results in a high percentage of that muscle's fibers being contracted.

All athletes consciously and unconsciously use pre-stretching in some fashion to their advantage. Take the baseball hitter who backswings before hitting the ball, or the boxer who draws back his fist before a punch, or the shot putter who gets that little dip before he throws.

Pre-stretching can also be used effectively in strength training sessions. Practiced properly, the technique will help you to handle heavier weights and thus bring into action a greater percentage of muscle mass during each repetition.

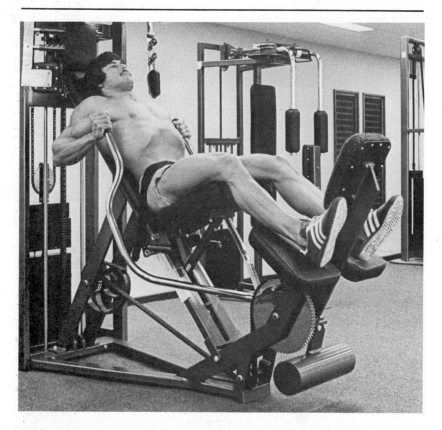

The pre-stretched position of the secondary movement on the double chest machine.

There is a thin line, however, between pre-stretching a muscle in the starting position of an exercise and following through with the repetition in the proper manner; and pre-stretching a muscle in the starting position and throwing the resistance. The key points to remember are pre-stretch, move quickly, then slow down.

The resistance should be lowered from the contracted position slowly and steadily until the resistance arm is about one inch from the position of full stretch. At that point, there should be a very quick twitch or thrust. After the quick twitch, the movement should be slowed down. The only time the resistance arm should be moved quickly is during the last one-quarter of the lowering (negative) part of the repetition and the first one-quarter to one-half of the raising (positive) part of the repetition. The last half of each repetition should always be performed smoothly.

REPETITIVE PRE-STRETCHING

Q. *Should pre-stretching be used on every repetition?*

A. If you're only interested in strength, the answer is yes. If you're also interested in flexibility, the answer is no.

Pre-stretching is necessary for maximum increases in strength. Thus a trainee must move quickly at the start of the movement to involve a greater number of muscle fibers in the contraction.

Pre-stretching, however, is not necessary in obtaining greater flexibility. What is needed is slow, relaxed movements that accentuate stretching rather than pre-stretching. The quick movements that are necessary in pre-stretching actually cause a muscle to contract rather than relax.

The ideal way to integrate both stretching for flexibility and pre-stretching for strength into a set of 10 repetitions is as follows:

During the first 3 or 4 repetitions, the trainee should emphasize the stretching part of each repetition. These repetitions should be performed slightly slower than normal. During the last 3 or 4 repetitions he should emphasize the pre-stretching part of the movement. These repetitions should be performed slightly faster than normal. The middle repetitions should be done with equal attention given to both stretching and pre-stretching.

NEGATIVE WORK

Q. *For strength-training purposes, why is negative work more productive than positive work?*

A. When you lift a resistance, your muscles are performing

positive work. Negative work is produced when you lower a weight.

A close examination of negative work reveals that it is the most important part of not only strength training, but a wide variety of other types of training.

First, pre-stretching, the neurological stimulation required for a high intensity of muscular contraction, comes from negative work. Exercises performed for the purpose of building strength are of very little value without high intensity of work.

Second, negative work reduces your reserve strength better than other methods of training. You can always continue to lower a resistance after you can no longer raise it. This allows you to reach a higher degree of high-intensity work.

Third, full-range exercise designed to work the entire length of a muscle also requires negative work. Negative work provides the back pressure of force that is required in a finishing position of full-muscular contraction.

Fourth, stretching is simply impossible without the back pressure provided by negative work. Thus exercises performed for the purpose of flexibility would be of little use without negative work.

Fifth, negative work makes it possible to exercise a muscle that is too weak to move against even the slightest amount of positive resistance. Thus negative work is a very valuable tool for the purpose of working muscles that have become weak as a result of injury.

It should be obvious that if you're concerned about strength, flexibility, or full-range exercise, you should pay close attention to the negative part of all exercises.

TRAINING EXPECTATIONS

Q. *What can a typical man expect from a Nautilus program?*

A. Some physiologists say that the typical, untrained man has the potential to increase his muscular strength approximately 300 percent. In reality, however, most men rarely get past the level of doubling their strength because they do not understand recovery ability.

While the typical man has the potential to increase his strength 300 percent, he can only increase his recovery ability about 50 percent. The stronger he becomes, the less exercise he needs.

Most trainees assume that the stronger they get the more exercise they need. But when they reach a certain level of strength they need shorter periods of harder exercise and longer periods of rest.

A hypothetical example should make this obvious. First, an individual's strength is tested to determine the amount of

Hypothetical example of changing exercise needs as strength increases. The weights given are averages of those used for all the exercises being done at a given time.

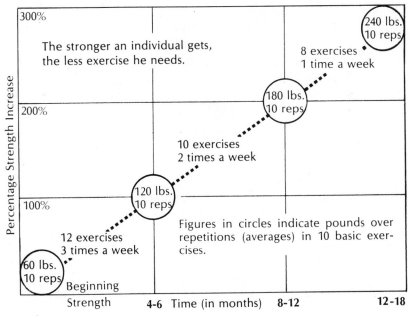

Maximum Strength Potential

Percentage Strength Increase

300%

The stronger an individual gets, the less exercise he needs.

8 exercises
1 time a week

240 lbs.
10 reps

180 lbs.
10 reps

200%

10 exercises
2 times a week

120 lbs.
10 reps

100%

Figures in circles indicate pounds over repetitions (averages) in 10 basic exercises.

12 exercises
3 times a week

60 lbs.
10 reps

Beginning
Strength   4-6   Time (in months)   8-12   12-18

weight he can lift for 10 repetitions, on 10 basic exercises. The results of this initial testing show he can do 60 pounds on the average of each exercise. Thus, his starting level is 60/10 (see graph).

Assuming he trains properly, he can expect to double his strength in 4 to 6 months, triple his strength in 8 to 12 months, and quadruple his strength in 12 to 18 months.

It is possible for this individual to reach his potential strength level in 12 to 18 months if he trains properly and if he understands his recovery ability.

Initially, almost any type of Nautilus training program will produce increases in strength for several months, simply because it is harder work than the average man is used to doing. The average man, at first, is not strong enough to make very deep inroads into his recovery ability. There is a vast difference between the recovery period of a 60-pound strength level and the 120-pound strength level.

In progressing from the 60-pound level to the 120-pound level, you should perform about 12 exercises, every other day, or three times per week. The 120-pound level is a critical point. Now you're strong enough to use up your recovery ability.

To progresss to the 180-pound level, you're going to have to train less. You must reduce your exercises from 12 to 10, and reduce your hard training days from three times to two a week.

Further progression from the 180-pound level to the 240-pound level necessitates additional reductions from 10 exercises to 8 exercises, and from two hard training days a week to one hard training day a week. The chart on the preceding page summarizes these details.

FREQUENCY

Q. *After a person doubles his strength, he should only train twice a week. Is that correct?*

A. The individual should still train three times a week, but only two of these workouts would be high intensity. He would train hard on Mondays and Fridays and medium on Wednesdays. The medium workout consists of the same exercises and resistance as the hard workout, but the medium exercise is ended two or three repetitions sooner. The medium workout does not stimulate growth, but it does prevent strength losses. It does not use up as much of the trainee's recovery ability as a hard workout.

It should be obvious that the muscular structure cannot grow without recovery ability. No amount of stimulation will produce growth if the body cannot supply the requirements for that growth.

It is important for the trainee to remember that the stronger he gets, the less exercise he needs.

POTENTIAL

Q. The chart on page 147 seems to indicate that if a trainee can perform 10 repetitions with 240 pounds on a certain exercise, he has reached his full potential. Is this correct?

A. No! The chart referred to is just a hypothetical example. In the chart, 240/10 represents the average of 10 different exercises after the trainee has quadrupled his strength. For example, using four Nautilus machines, he might be able to train with 275 pounds on the hip and back, 225 on the leg press, 180 on the pullover, and 100 on the biceps curl. The average of these four exercises would be 195 pounds.

Naturally, an individual will be able to increase the strength of some muscle groups faster and to a greater degree than others. Much of this depends on his bodily proportions, neurological efficiency, and the size of the muscle mass that he is working.

The typical, untrained man should be able to quadruple his overall strength, if he works out properly.

TYPICAL MAN

Q. *What is a "typical" man?*

A. According to the U.S. government, the average man in this country is 5'10" in height, weighs 154 pounds, and is 28 years of age. With the proper training, the average man should be able to quadruple his strength. Most men fall in this category. Some men may be able to quintuple their strength; others may be able only to triple their strength. A very few men have the potential to be exceptionally strong, almost to a super-human degree. And there are other men that have very little potential for strength. But, generally speaking, most men have the potential to quadruple their strength.

SUPERVISION

Q. *What does an athlete do when there is no coach available to supervise his training?*

A. The athlete should find a training partner. They then push each other one at a time through a hard workout. After several weeks of training, both athletes should have learned enough about each other to organize productive training sessions.

PARTIAL REPETITIONS

Q. *On a Nautilus machine, if a person cannot complete a full range of movement after about 8 repetitions, should he continue to do partial repetitions until failure?*

A. The answer to this question depends on the Nautilus machine being used. On the single-joint rotary movements, such as the pullover, leg extension, and leg curl, the cams are about 90-percent efficient at working the desired muscle. Partial repetitions should *not* be done on the single-joint machines. Doing so means a disproportionate emphasis on part of the movement, since the cam is designed to work the muscle proportionally.

With the multiple-joint exercises, such as the leg press, overhead press, and pulldown, partial repetitions at the end of a set may be advantageous. Multiple-joint exercises on Nautilus machines are about 25-percent efficient. It is impossible to attain a proper full-range strength curve on such a movement, so partial repetitions are called for.

EXCESSIVE FACIAL EXPRESSION

Q. *What is so bad about "making faces" or excessive facial expression during Nautilus training?*

A. Any time you "make a face," you must contract many small muscles of the face and neck. Not only does this take a certain amount of energy, but it also reduces your ability to contract larger muscle groups repeatedly.

If you were trying to determine how much weight you

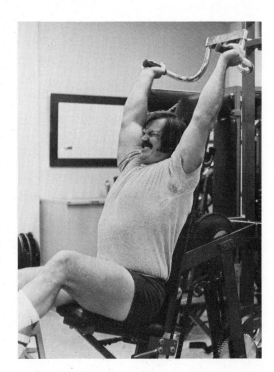

For best results from Nautilus training, contraction of the facial muscles should be kept to a minimum.

could handle for a maximum-attempt-one-repetition effort,
it might be beneficial to scream and shout and make faces.
But unless you were a competitive weightlifter, there is no
need to try to determine how much weight you can handle
for one repetition.

In performing 8 to 12 repetitions of a dozen different
exercises, it reduces your efficiency to make faces. If you are
using the leg extension machine, you should concentrate on
the quadriceps muscles as you perform the exercise, and at
the same time, try to relax the non-involved muscles of your
body. Bringing into play the facial or other upper body
muscles forces your transport system to do a less efficient
job on the legs.

Making faces convinces you, as well as your instructor,
that you are working harder than you actually are. This
reaction can stop you short of momentary muscular failure
on many exercises.

Furthermore, making faces unnecessarily elevates the
blood pressure. Forceful gripping of the hands also increases
blood pressure to dangerously high levels. Since high-
intensity exercise by itself elevates your blood pressure
temporarily, there is no need to make it higher by making
faces or excessive gripping.

For better results from Nautilus exercise, you must learn to
relax the muscles of your face, neck, and hands as well as
other muscles that are not involved in the specific movement.

PRE-EXHAUSTION PRINCIPLE

Q. On the Nautilus double shoulder machine, should the
seat be readjusted after the lateral raise in order to provide a
greater range of movement in the overhead press? If so,
why?

A. You should make sure the seat on the double shoulder
machine is raised very quickly. A muscle can recover 50
percent of its exhausted strength in about three seconds. For

best results, you should move from the lateral raise to the overhead press in less than three seconds.

All Nautilus double machines (compound leg, pullover/ torso arm, behind neck/torso arm, double chest and double shoulder) were designed to make use of the pre-exhaustion principle. The purpose of this principle is to pre-exhaust a muscle group by performing a single-joint exercise that involves specific muscles. This is immediately followed by a multiple-joint exercise that brings into play other surrounding muscles to force the pre-exhausted muscles to work even harder.

The primary exercise of the double shoulder machine, the lateral raise, is a single-joint movement that works the deltoids without involving the arms. The secondary exercise, the overhead press, is a multiple-joint movement that involves the deltoids and the arms. Done back to back, the overhead press uses the strength of the triceps to force the pre-exhausted deltoids to work even harder.

One of the problems with exercise for the torso muscles is that these large muscles are stronger than the bending or straightening muscles of the arms. As a result, in conventional exercise, the arms always tire before the torso muscles are exhausted. The arms are the weak link in working the torso. This problem is overcome if the torso muscles are first pre-exhausted with an exercise that only indirectly involves the arms. In less than three seconds, the primary exercise is followed by a multiple-joint exercise for the torso muscles and the arms. Thus the arms, which are now temporarily stronger than the pre-exhausted torso muscles, can be used to force these torso muscles to reach a deeper state of exhaustion.

MOTIVATION

Q. *Is there a best way to keep athletes motivated toward Nautilus training?*

A. There are many motivational techniques that can be

used successfully. Any way that athletes, individually or collectively, can be motivated to an optimal extent is the best way. It takes a sensitive coach to be aware of the needs of his athletes and to know the motivational techniques that inspire them to do their best.

If a coach is in doubt about which method to use, a true story from the history books may help him decide.

Over 400 years ago, in the Andes Mountains of South America, there lived a tribe of Indians called the Incas. One day, the leader of the tribe told his workers that he wanted a monument in his honor erected on top of a nearby mountain. To make this monument more spectacular, the leader wanted huge boulders from the valley moved to the top of the mountain.

After several days of work, the foreman of the slave laborers reported to the leader with a problem:

"The trail to the top of the mountain is very narrow and winding," said the foreman. "Only 100 men are able to grasp the rope that is attached to the largest boulder. One hundred men cannot pull that boulder up the mountain. It should remain in the valley."

"No," countered the leader. "The largest boulder must be pulled to the top, and I'll tell you how to do it. Go back to the work camp and kill 50 of the 100 men that were involved in the first attempt. Then command the remaining men to pull the boulder to the top."

The next day, the confused foreman brought the same problem back to the leader. "The boulder has not budged. If 100 men could not pull the boulder up the mountain, certainly 50 can't. The largest boulder should remain in the valley."

"Never!" shouted the leader. "Return to the work camp and this time kill 25 of the 50 men."

The remaining 25 men, so the story goes, successfully pulled the largest boulder to the top of the mountain.

Fear, according to many historians, is the world's greatest motivator.

While coaches cannot use the same approach that the Incan leader used, they can employ a healthy fear, a fear that commands respect and esteem; a fear that, if used properly, will produce better Nautilus training results from all athletes.

GAINING BULK

Q. *Is it possible to gain bulk using Nautilus equipment?*

A. The word "bulk" is misleading. The two most change-able components of the human body are muscle and fat. Gaining bulk to most athletes and coaches means adding body weight; and body weight comes from getting fatter by eating more calories. Gaining fat makes an athlete slower, less coordinated, less healthy, and more prone to heart and other diseases in his later life.

Training on Nautilus equipment does not significantly alter fat cells or fat storage depots. Nautilus training, however, if it is performed properly, will significantly increase an athlete's muscle mass. Athletes should be motivated to gain muscle, not fat. Muscle is gained by proper strength training, not excessive calories.

LOSING FAT

Q. *How does Nautilus contribute to a fat-loss program?*

A. Nautilus contributes to a fat loss program in two ways:

1. Since Nautilus involves full-range exercise and no other activity does, common sense shows that training on Nautilus equipment burns more calories than any similar activity. As a rough estimate, walking briskly requires 5.2 calories per minute, bicycling consumes 8.6 calories per minute, jogging takes 10 calories a minute, and swimming uses up 11.2 calories per minute. Properly performed, Nautilus exercise, depending on the machine used, burns between 15 and 20 calories per minute.

2. Nautilus increases muscular size, and larger muscles

require more calories at rest and work. The more muscle an individual has on his body, the more calories this individual requires each day.

Thus, using Nautilus equipment provides a double-reducing effect. The body requires calories to be burned during Nautilus exercise, and additional calories as a result of the produced growth.

DEVELOPING QUICKNESS

Q. *Can training on Nautilus improve an athlete's quickness?*

A. Quickness is a product of many factors, some of which are as follows: (1) the amount of muscle on the body, (2) the amount of fat, (3) the muscle mass to body weight ratio, (4) skill, (5) bodily proportions, and (6) motivation.

The easiest way to accelerate the athlete's quickness is to increase his muscle mass, which will favorably change his ratio of muscle mass to body weight. The most effective way to accomplish this is Nautilus training combined with a low-calorie, well-balanced diet.

CASEY VIATOR

Q. *Didn't Casey Viator gain most of his muscular size and strength from barbells?*

A. Casey did train several years on conventional equipment prior to meeting Arthur Jones in 1970. His best training results, however, came during the several months that preceded the 1971 Mr. America contest. Arthur Jones personally supervised each of his workouts.

The important thing to remember about Casey is that he had the genetic potential to be big and strong before he ever got interested in training. Almost any type of resistance exercise—gymnastics, barbells, Universal, or Nautilus—would have given him results. He inherited extremely long muscle bellies. Actual measurements show that Casey has four times as much muscular mass potential as the average American male.

Arthur Jones makes it a point to tell bodybuilders who visit the Nautilus headquarters that Casey has a sister with similar potential who weighs a solid 180 pounds. And she has never done any resistance training.

BODYBUILDING AND NAUTILUS

Q. *Why don't the well-known bodybuilders, other than Casey Viator, use Nautilus equipment?*

A. Several well-known bodybuilders do use Nautilus, but they are exceptions to the rule. Most bodybuilders are addicted to long, low-intensity workouts. They claim to train

Mr. Universe of 1978, Mike Mentzer is a firm believer in Nautilus high-intensity training. Mike's brother Ray, the current Mr. America, also uses Nautilus equipment.

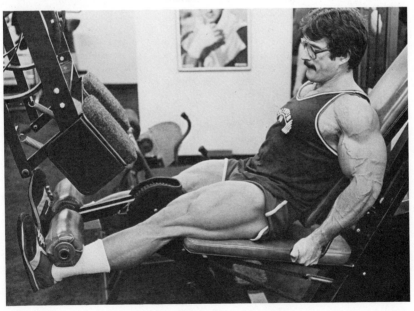

for best results, but in reality there are multiple other reasons that are interwoven into their training beliefs and behaviors.

Generally speaking, competitive bodybuilding is physical, mental, and social. Most bodybuilders subconsciously put it in the mental and social realm rather than the physical where it belongs. There are the sights and smells of the gym; the rituals of training and looking into mirrors, such as getting a muscular pump and keeping it for an extended period of time; the socialization that takes place between trainees; and the entire atmosphere that surrounds the bodybuilding world.

It is difficult to convince a bodybuilder who has been training for years in the conventional fashion that he can get several times better results from training with Nautilus equipment. Even if he is convinced about the effectiveness of Nautilus, this only makes inroads into one of the multiple reasons behind why he is exercising. It is similar to recommending that a person open a completely physiological restaurant where he would test, evaluate, and feed his customers according to their actual needs. He would learn quickly that people do not eat to satisfy their physical requirements. They eat out of habit, out of desire to be sociable, and many other reasons. The same factors are at work in the bodybuilder's habits and behaviors.

Nautilus equipment is definitely the best way to body-build. It is the only equipment in existence that is designed around the physiological requirements of the human body. In order to get the best results from Nautilus, however, the psychological and social aspects of training have to be de-emphasized. The basis of training must be physiological. Nautilus must be performed slower, harder, and briefer, and not in a party atmosphere.

TRAINING MORE

Q. *What happens when a person performs more than 12*

Nautilus exercises during a workout or trains more than three times a week?

A. When either of these things happens, and they frequently do, it is obvious that the individual is not training in a high-intensity fashion. It is also obvious that he is not interested in obtaining the best possible results from Nautilus.

Without at least one high-intensity workout a week, it is difficult to maintain a level of fitness. It usually takes two high-intensity sessions per week to increase one's level of fitness.

To exercise in a low-intensity fashion is not all bad. It does burn a few calories and provides the trainee with some activity. But it just as certainly does not produce anything close to the physiological stimulation that a small amount of high-intensity exercise would produce.

THE BEST FITNESS ACTIVITY

Q. *Many exercise authorities have stated that the activity which provides the athlete with the most fitness in the least amount of time is running. Why does Nautilus disagree with this concept?*

A. A well-rounded fitness activity should do at least four things: (1) build balanced muscular strength, (2) increase joint flexibility, (3) improve cardiovascular endurance, and (4) reduce injuries.

Running builds very little strength, and the strength it does build is not balanced. Running does absolutely nothing for flexibility. Most runners lose flexibility in their lower body because they use predominantly mid-range contractions. Running can develop high levels of cardiovascular endurance, if the running is done properly. But the risk of subjecting the body to excessive pounding may not be worth the cardiovascular benefits. Each time the foot hits the ground the body absorbs a force of two to five times the runner's body weight. Recent statistics show that there is an 80-percent probability of injury from one year of regular running. Thus, running only fulfills one of the four criteria above. It improves cardiovascular endurance while doing nothing for balanced muscular strength and flexibility, and it contributes to a host of injuries.

The best all-around fitness activity, the activity that provides the athlete or the non-athlete with the most exercise in the least amount of time, is Nautilus training. Nautilus training, if it is done properly, improves strength, endurance, flexibility, and reduces the probability of injury.

ONE SET VERSUS MULTIPLE SETS

Q. *Why is performing only one set of a given Nautilus machine better than three to four sets?*

A. Arthur Jones uses the following analogy concerning the performance of multiple sets: "It takes only one properly placed shot to kill a rabbit, or an elephant. Additional shots will serve no purpose except unnecessary destruction of the meat. The same is true of exercise."

If one set of a properly performed exercise will stimulate a muscle to grow, additional sets are counter-productive because they use up valuable recovery ability without contributing to further growth.

HIGHER REPETITIONS

Q. *Would it be better to perform 15 to 20 repetitions, or 8 to 12 on the Nautilus leg machines>*

A. Repetitions are not as important as time. Skeletal muscle strength is produced by working with the anaerobic metabolic processes. The anaerobic metabolic processes are best taxed by intensive exercise that lasts at least 30 seconds, but not more than 70 seconds. Continuing an exercise past 70 seconds may involve the aerobic processes, or heart and lungs, to a greater degree than the skeletal muscles. A repetition correctly performed on a Nautilus machine, depending on the range of movement, takes from 3 to 8 seconds. If a typical repetition takes about 6 seconds to perform, simple multiplication reveals that 8 repetitions would equal 48 seconds, and 12 repetitions would equal 72 seconds.

Eight to 12 repetitions, or 30 to 70 seconds, apply to all Nautilus machines. If a trainee rests for several seconds when the weight stack touches, or rests in the lock-out position of a multiple-joint exercise, more than 12 repetitions will be possible. Each time there is a slight rest period, the working muscles temporarily recover. For example, 15 to 20 repetitions could be performed o the leg press since most trainees eventually learn to rest in the lock-out position. Or 15 to 20 repetitions might be performed on the calf raise since it involves such a short range of movement. Eight to 12 repetitions, given that there is little or no rest between movements, seem to be the best guideline for trainees to follow in using all Nautilus machines.

NAUTILUS AND OTHER ACTIVITIES

Q. *What should an individual who likes to combine Nautilus training with sports such as running or racquetball do for best results?*

A. Under ideal conditions, you would run or play racquetball in the morning and Nautilus-train in the afternoon. There should be about four hours' time lapse between both activities, with a complete day's rest afterward. Thus, you might play racquetball for an hour at 11:00 A.M., eat a light lunch at 12:30 P.M., and train on Nautilus machines around 4:00 or 5:00 P.M. The following day you would rest, relax, and recover. An every-other-day schedule like that produces the best combined results.

Most people, however, because of the inconvenience of training twice in one day, would rather run or play racquetball on one day and use Nautilus on the next. Or they will try to do both activities on the same day with only a brief rest in between. Neither of these methods has proved to be superior in results to the first discussed method.

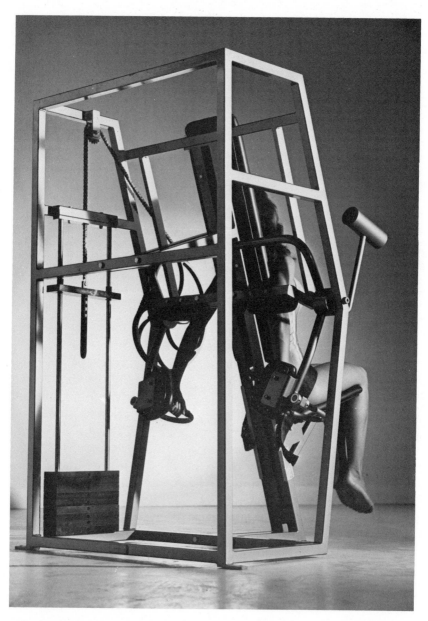

Compound position triceps machine

CHAPTER THIRTEEN

the future of nautilus

In 1976, an 8,000 square foot orthopedic clinic was built on Nautilus property in Lake Helen. Within the first year alone, over 100 surgical procedures were performed on injured athletes. Each was rehabilitated on Nautilus equipment with a 100 percent success rate.

The primary goal of sports medicine is not the rehabilitation but the prevention of injuries. Nautilus is most concerned about conditioning the human body as a means of improving performance and preventing injury. It should be recognized, however, that the same principles that are used for conditioning purposes can also be used to rehabilitate injured parts of the body.

One of the biggest Nautilus success stories was baseball player Eric Soderholm. On May 8, 1976, Dr. Fred L. Allman and Dr. James D. Key performed surgery on Eric's left knee. Dr. Allman noted after the operation that Eric's chances of playing professional baseball again were less than 50-50.

163

Rehabilitation of an injured limb is aided by training of the uninjured body parts in a high-intensity fashion. This prevents much of the atrophy that would normally occur to the injured limb and the body.

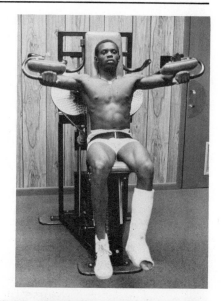

For rehabilitation purposes, weak limbs can be strengthened by training each leg, or arm, separately. Eric Soderholm is shown performing a leg press.

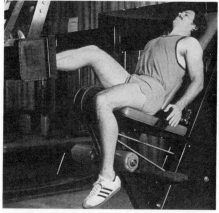

After spending eight months of rehabilitation and training at the Nautilus clinic in Florida, Eric returned to spring training in 1977 almost three times as strong as in any previous year. He had his best season ever and as a result was voted the American League's Comeback Player of the Year.

A book was written describing Soderholm's remarkable

recovery, and Nautilus produced a 12-minute film that covers his surgery and rehabilitation. Both have met wide acceptance in the medical community. The production of diagnostic, surgical, and rehabilitation films on all aspects of sports medicine are goals that Nautilus is achieving at this moment.

One of the general health problems is the difficulty in distinguishing between the physiological and psychological effects of a given treatment or program.

The placebo effect is a recognized phenomenon in medical drug testing. It may be defined as what happens when there is a change in the status of an illness which cannot be attributed to a chemically active substance upon an organism. Sugar pills often produce the same effect on humans as do strong drugs.

The enthusiasm and expectations that doctors and patients may share for a new course of treatment is fully recognized by medical researchers. This same type of enthusiasm and expectancy can be used to explain why some athletes are so convinced that they are affected by particular training routines, habits, and beliefs. Dr. George Sheehan goes as far as to say that the faith individuals place in a remedy or routine can produce improvement in 60–70 percent of the cases.

In the physiological realm, many things are unpredictable. This problem stems from the fact that few tools are available which can reliably measure physiological parameters. Throughout physiology literature, there are numerous references to measurements of strength, flexibility, cardiovascular endurance, and percentage of body fat. Yet a thorough examination of the mechanical tools used to measure these parameters reveals that they are not trustworthy. Quality control in the manufacture of these tools is virtually nonexistent. The directions for use are scanty. Calibration is next to impossible.

This does not stop an increasing amount of research that is published widely in scientific journals. But few people ever

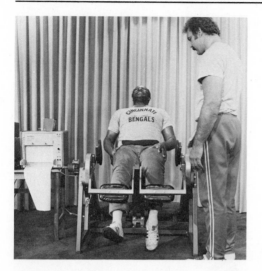

Nautilus will soon be producing a complete line of physiological testing machines. Here, Dick Butkus tests the strength of a football player's quadriceps. This is a static test being performed in one of nine possible positions.

consider the question, "What if the tools are not accurate?"

Nautilus Sports/Medical Industries plans to build tools that will accurately measure flexibility, cardiovascular endurance, percentage of body fat, and muscular strength at any position throughout a full range of movement. Then at least the initial stages of meaningful research in exercise physiology will be possible.

Such tools will also make it possible for physicians to prescribe exact amounts of exercise. More important, however, is the fact that instant feedback will be available to the physician, therapist, and patient. The exercise machine of the future will not eliminate "cheating" in exercise, but it will make it possible for those involved to know when, where, and how they are performing the movement. All of this will be done with the aid of a computer.

The trainee enters the sports medicine center of the future, pulls his pre-programmed plastic card out of the file

A prototype of a computerized Nautilus biceps ma-
chine. The monitor in front
of the trainee provides in-
struction, pacing, and immediate feedback for each
repetition.

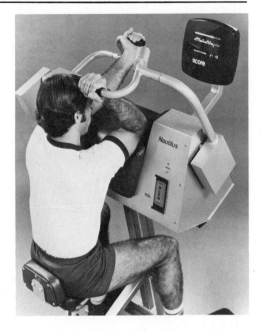

and inserts it into a slot in a computerized Nautilus machine.
As soon as the individual's card is inserted, his number will
appear on the appropriate machine. This machine will be
automatically set for the trainee with careful consideration
for such things as existing strength level, degree of flexibility,
cardiovascular endurance, age, and previous medical history.
From that moment on, a monitor on each machine will tell
the trainee what to do, how to do it, how hard to do it, and
how often to do it. And the machine will keep a permanent
record of what is actually done. The level of resistance will
be whatever the trainee requires at that point. Naturally, this
will be pre-determined by the physician or therapist.

The computerized machines of the future will not make
the individual exercise properly. Nothing can do that. All
that anybody or anything can do is make it possible for an
individual to exercise properly, and then encourage him to
do it. The machine will tell him when what he is doing is

right, and when it is wrong. The machine can do all of those things, and do them better than any human supervisor.

The machines will do many things that no human can. They will preserve an exact record of the trainee's actual workouts, and the computer will automatically and instantly change the workouts when needed. Sensing and reacting to any reasonable number of physiological factors, the machine will offer a degree of safety not possible before.

What will be the results of such exercise? Any kind and degree of results that can now be produced by any type of exercise will be possible:

Increased strength
Increased flexibility
Increased cardiovascular endurance
Rehabilitation following certain types of illness
Programs designed to maintain fitness

The future Nautilus machines can be computer-programmed for any purpose. But perhaps of greatest importance, a machine will not lose interest in the subjects working under its supervision.

Motivation seems to be the most pressing problem in physical fitness. It is difficult to induce people to perform exercise properly. If both the form and intensity of work are proper, exercise is capable of producing surprising results in a short span of time. But there seems to be a natural tendency to permit a rapid deterioration in the style of performance, and to gradually reduce the intensity of exercise without even being aware that such is occurring.

The design of most exercise equipment makes such problems almost inevitable. The problems are inherent, but they can be solved.

Poor form and lowered intensity result from a desire to show progress. Under the mistaken impression that they are improving at a faster rate, most people quickly start changing the form or intensity of exercise. They are encouraged by the fact that doing so increases the amount of resistance they can handle. But by that time they are throwing the weight, not lifting it.

No increase in resistance is meaningful unless the form remains unchanged, and no amount of exercise will be effective if the form is not good. Future computerized Nautilus equipment will take subjectivity out of training.

Dr. James A. Nicholas of New York, one of the nation's leaders in sports medicine, recently took a survey to find out how many places there are in the country calling themselves "sports medicine clinics." He found that there are at least 900. Only 50–75 of the 900 clinics, according to Dr. Nicholas, are run by people trained in medicine. As might be expected, there is little consistency in what is recommended or practiced from clinic to clinic.

A patient may find that an ankle sprain is treated with heat

A small section of one of the Nautilus television studios in Lake Helen, Florida.

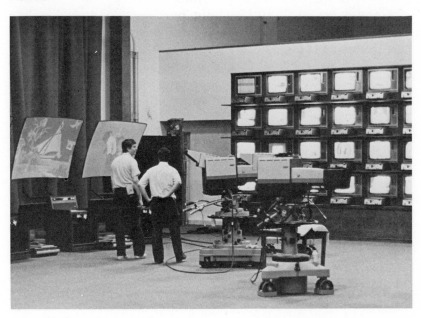

in Seattle and cold in Tampa. Runner's knee may be exercised in Dallas, but rested in Cleveland. An athlete may be strength-trained explosively in New York and told to move as slowly as possible in Los Angeles. While detailed, factual information exists on these and many sports medicine topics, the dissemination of this material is scanty.

But by the early 1980s, Nautilus will have developed full-scale television studios in the Lake Helen facility. The purpose of these studios will be education, not entertainment. The video disc will be the crucial tool in the dissemination of sports medicine information. The video disc looks like a thick, long-playing record and can be manufactured as cheaply. It has a visual component that is easily adapted to an average television set. It will be possible to sell a two-hour video disc for less than $5, when the same program on videotape might cost $100, and 16-millimeter film would cost $1,000 or more.

The video disc allows freeze-frame and slow-motion techniques never before possible. This technology will thus make it possible to study everything that moves, whether in the operating room, on the playing field, or in the fitness center.

Injuries that have previously been filmed can be studied to determine their cause. There will be opportunities to show films of a knee operation, the correct form to use while on Nautilus machines, a symposium on the prevention of neck injuries in football, or any of a growing library of Nautilus Sports/Medical films.

A satellite link with Lake Helen, Florida, will enable the Nautilus Network to beam shows throughout the world.

This communication potential, combined with the Nautilus computerized exercise machine, opens the doors for the much-needed consistency in procedures of rehabilitation, conditioning, and record keeping.

Nautilus, the symbol of geometric perfection, was reborn in the form of a machine which is revolutionizing exercise and sports medicine.

index